SOUND MIND ◆ SOUND BODY

SOUND MIND

◆

SOUND BODY

DAVID KIRSCH'S ULTIMATE
6-WEEK FITNESS TRANSFORMATION
FOR MEN AND WOMEN

DAVID KIRSCH

RODALE®

© 2002 by David Kirsch
Cover Photograph © by Shonna Valeska
Interior Photographs © by Shonna Valeska, except for food and exercise photos, which are by Mitch Mandel/Rodale Images

Printed in the United States of America
Rodale Inc. makes every effort to use acid-free ∞, recycled paper ♻.

Cover and Interior Designer: Christopher Rhoads
Hair and Makeup Stylists: Linda Fung, Colleen Kobrick-Kuehne, and Barbara Camp
Food Stylist: Diane Vezza
Prop Stylist: Janet Bowblis
Model: Stacy Curtis/Axis Models and Talent
Model's Clothing by Rogiani, Inc.

Library of Congress Cataloging-in-Publication Data
Kirsch, David.
  Sound mind, sound body : David Kirsch's ultimate 6-week fitness transformation for men and women / David Kirsch.
     p.   cm.
  ISBN 1–57954–450–9 hardcover
  1. Physical fitness.   2. Health.   I. Title.
  GV481 .K534   2002
  613.7—dc21   2001005877

Distributed to the book trade by St. Martin's Press

2   4   6   8   10   9   7   5   3   1   hardcover

Visit us on the Web at www.rodalestore.com, or call us toll-free at (800) 848-4735.

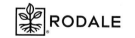

WE **INSPIRE** AND **ENABLE** PEOPLE TO IMPROVE
THEIR LIVES AND THE WORLD AROUND THEM

To Mom and Dad—
The journey begins with you.

CONTENTS

Foreword | ix

Introduction | xiii

Chapter One: Sound Beginnings | 1

Chapter Two: Sound Confidence | 15

Chapter Three: Sound Training | 27

Chapter Four: Sound Eating | 135

Chapter Five: Sound Thinking | 203

Chapter Six: Sound Living | 215

Acknowledgments | 235

FOREWORD

FOR THE LONGEST time, I'd been hearing about a trainer with a very special gift who was helping people transform their relationships to fitness, to health, to their bodies—in fact, to their lives. I'd also heard about this gem of a fitness club, the Madison Square Club, in the heart of New York City, where this trainer held court.

In the City, where the demand for quality in fitness training is coupled with a large pool of available talent, discrimination is key in finding the fitness club or individual that will help change your dreams of having a great bod into reality. Word of mouth passes quickly around town when a new course or trainer has surfaced with the latest and greatest thing to whip you into shape. They often fade just as quickly.

Then there is the endurance of David Kirsch, the Madison Square Club, and the fierce loyalty of his clients. With David, you have a man who describes himself as only "an ordinary guy from Long Island," to which I add, "with an extraordinary commitment to peoples' lives and well-being."

From events 15 years ago that forever transformed him, he re-created himself into the wellness trainer he is today. Some of the most beautiful people and most celebrated faces in modeling and show business seek out David for his talent, his precise manner of training, and his passion for a deeper result than just a pretty body. He seeks to envelop you in the substance of fitness that includes every element of wellness: your diet, your emotional life, how you deal with stress, and your spirituality, a component that so often is neglected.

There is responsibility that comes with carrying the mantle of fitness guru, and it's evident in all the things to which David is committed. When you look beyond the celebrities that come to him, you'll see the people that come to him striving for a better life. Where the grind of life has bled the spirit out of them, they are reawakened to the joy and fun of being fit and its necessity in staying competitive in today's world. Good sense and a good workout are his keys for opening you to the benefits of exercise as a necessary component for a great life.

To be competitive in today's world, to make sure you stay in the game of life, you need a winning formula. To dismiss the role of exercise or nutrition is to do so at your own peril, when so much may be at stake. We live in times when to deal with the demands and obligations of our lives, we have no choice but to be fit. We need sound advice and the motivational approach that fits with our lives.

In this book, David carefully outlines for you the elements that will allow you to experience the results he produces at the Madison Square Club, whether you're at home or at your local fitness club. In all the years I've worked in the arena of human development and well-being, I've met few people that offer such a full package. In fact, I would more accurately call it a pathway to successful living through a lifetime of fitness.

David's formula combines the knowledge and information you need to look and feel your best. With the many voices and approaches to health you're likely to hear, this one is distinguished by its authenticity and the rigor of its veracity: The results he gets with his legions of devoted clients speak for themselves. If you want the magic and mystique that people seek with David Kirsch, you'll find it here in this exceptional book.

You've heard it a million times: the platitudes, the overblown recommendations to follow one diet or exercise plan that often lead to disappointment when their promised quick solutions don't work. With David Kirsch, you must bring commitment to the table.

In the process of blending his knowledge with your commitment, you'll hammer out the body you've always wanted. Make no mistake, you have to earn this body. But with David Kirsch, you have the means to achieve it through an extremely thoughtful and well-developed exercise and nutritional program. Wherever you are and wherever you live, you can incorporate these principles that are guided by excellence and will

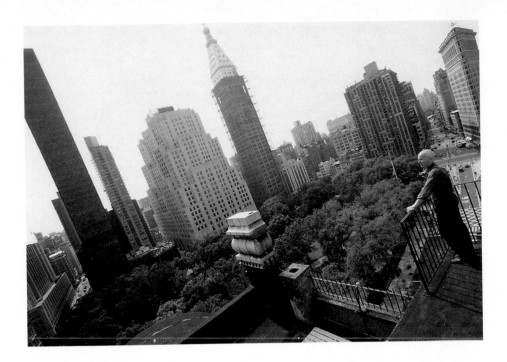

infuse you with optimism as you experience results.

You may never achieve the body of a supermodel (guess which ones work with David?), but with this book, you can certainly achieve the best body God gave you. I am proud to call David my ally and fellow warrior for well-being.

—Oz Garcia, Montauk, New York
June 2001

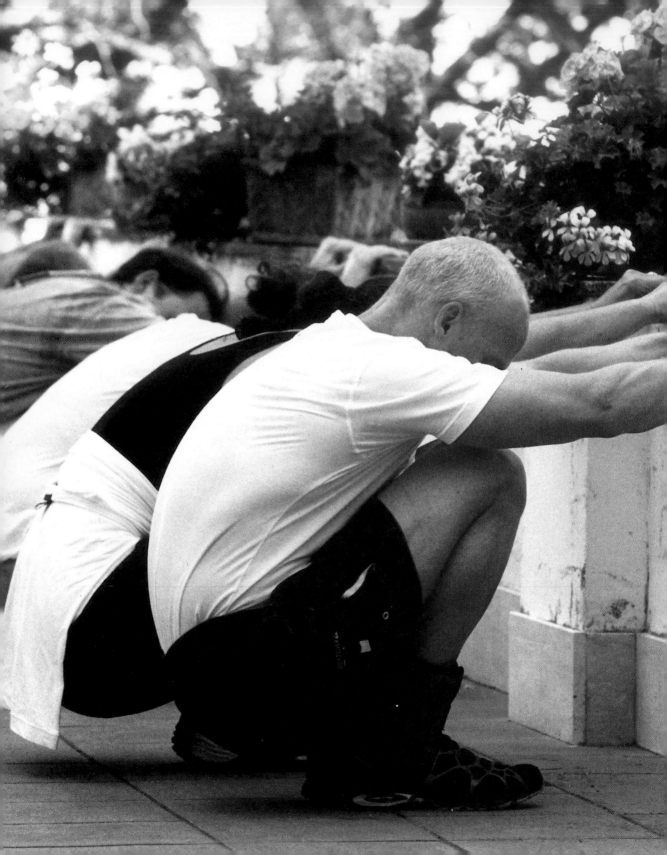

INTRODUCTION

SOUND MIND, Sound Body—the balance of the physical, mental, and spiritual lies at the core of my program.

After 15 years of personal training, and longer than that in researching and experiencing different fitness trends, nutritional guideline books, and self-proclaimed healing and get-well books, I have decided that it is time to speak out. There is a way to reach the perfect balance of mind, body, and spirit. I call that balance Sound Mind, Sound Body. The integral elements necessary in attaining a Sound Mind, Sound Body require finding the balance among a) proper workouts, b) nutritious foods, and c) a spiritual and emotional balance that in part relies on the successful completion of a) and b).

I used to attribute the saying "what doesn't kill us makes us stronger" to my mother's sagelike wisdom. But despite my incorrect attribution, those words have helped transform me from an undecided, unhappy, and unfulfilled litigator into the directed, highly motivated successful owner of the Madison Square Club, New York City's premier private training facility.

The strength and courage imbued in me by my parents from an early age gave me the inner strength and fortitude to withstand the growing pains and mistakes of my twenties. I was quick to realize that there was a reason for everything in this world. If one stood back and didn't react to situations but rather reflected and acted calmly, most potential problems were surmountable.

The metamorphosis from lawyer to entrepreneur was a painstaking one, filled with many angst-ridden moments. But after 5 years as a litigator and general practitioner battling daily migraines caused by the stresses of my career, I realized that I had another calling. I was meant to be what I now term a Wellness Trainer.

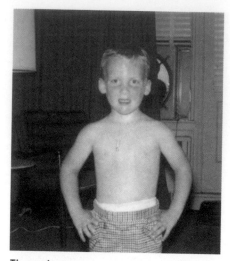

The early years

THE BACKGROUND

Now, before you start rolling your eyes and thinking, "This guy is a fitness and nutrition zealot who has never been out of shape a day in his life," think again. I grew up a skinny kid who possessed average physical skills. My adolescent school years were actually quite tortuous. I remember elementary and junior high school gym classes with dread. I was one of those kids who couldn't inch even a few feet up the rope that every school gym seems to have hanging from the ceiling. I just didn't have any natural athletic talent, or so I thought. You might identify with the memories of those painful times.

At the same time, I grew up watching my dad work out religiously. His training room was his refuge from all the frustrations and stresses of the

day. Although he tried to convince me to find my haven in physical fitness, it wasn't until I discovered running in my early twenties that it all started to make sense to me. Once I started, I was a total convert—working out and being healthy and physically active would become second nature and the response to all that ailed me. All of my dad's teachings came back to me. As is often true, everything comes full circle; I finally embraced and understood his passion for fitness.

I see my transformed body as a symbol of my transformed life. When I was younger, I had not only an unhealthy body but also an unhealthy mind. My lack of self-esteem and self-worth held me back and prevented me from realizing my true potential. I aimlessly drifted about pursuing ambiguous dreams. I ended up in law school, chasing after prestige, but prestige didn't satisfy my soul.

Through much trial and error, I eventually discovered my true calling: training people to reach their full physical and psychological potential. The process of discovery from attorney to Wellness Trainer was filled with years of anxiety and personal trauma. I went through many dark periods, especially after I lost my uncle, aunt, and best friend to sudden terminal illnesses. It took mental, physical, and emotional work for me to emerge from that dark place, but once I did, I realized that I had discovered what I had been looking for all along: a Sound Mind and a Sound Body. I became evangelical in my desire to pass that discovery on to others. It became my life's calling.

Through my techniques as a Wellness Trainer, I have been able to turn even the most reluctant of couch potatoes into fitness and nutrition enthusiasts. After reading this book, I want you to feel calmer and more focused in a positive direction about life, love, and pursuits of physical, mental, and spiritual happiness. Ultimately, this book will help you achieve your goals when nothing before has worked. The transformation will be life-altering.

THE PROGRAM

I don't believe in diets. I don't believe in diet pills. They don't address the reason one needs to lose weight or start an intensive exercise program in the first place. Diets and diet pills are bandages—they treat the symptom but not the cause. And I'm not the answer or the cure either, but rather the prescription that can set you on the right path. Through personal stories, anecdotes, and client testimonials, you will see that although the road may be bumpy at times, it is, in the end, ultimately navigable.

The key to reaching your goals lies in Soundness. You must eat, exercise, and think Soundly. You can't separate those elements. Soundness is what creates the radiance that I mentioned earlier. It's what creates personal satisfaction. It's what makes all the pieces of your life fit together. This program is a complete mind-body package. My Sound Mind, Sound Body program is a series of six steps along a lifelong path to wellness.

Sound beginnings. Many people sabotage their wellness habits from the start by rushing head first into a new fitness pursuit. But a little planning—before you start exercising or changing your eating habits—will help you stick to your new habits for the long term. Chapter 1 will tell you everything you need to know about joining a gym, setting up your home gym, hiring a trainer, finding time for exercise, and more.

Sound confidence. The importance of reasonable goal setting cannot be underestimated. When you bought this book, you probably had a goal. Maybe it was to lose 10 pounds or to firm up your rear end. To help you stay motivated to meet that goal, you need to break it down into small, measurable steps so that you'll see results every single week. I'll show you how to do that and more in chapter 2. We also will address five different body types—the apple, pear, stick, round, and fit persons, and their relative body issues. Each has particular needs and, consequently, different goals.

Sound training. In chapter 3, we get to the meat of your fitness transformation. Unlike other fitness plans, my program places a heavy emphasis on using your mind to direct your workout. I will show you the correct and incorrect ways to perform an exercise and tell you which muscles to engage. This type of Sound Training will keep you feeling motivated for years to come. It will also help you achieve results faster.

Sound eating. Take the word "diet" out of your vocabulary! You don't need a calculator or calorie counter to follow the Sound Eating program that I lay out in chapter 4. I don't believe you should spend your time figuring out the percentage of protein to carbohydrate to fat that you are eating. I do believe you should eat wholesome, fresh foods. There will be certain foods to avoid (starchy carbohydrates and sugary fruits), but I will show you how to make intelligent food choices without the feeling of deprivation and a negative sense of self. That's the most important change you need to make in order to see fast results. It may sound simple, but it works.

Sound thinking. To cement new eating and exercise habits, you need to change what's going on inside your head and within your life. The Sound Thinking that I propose in chapter 5 will not only help you carve the body you desire but also will help you in your career, your relationships, and your personal happiness.

Sound living. Chapter 6 will show you how to incorporate your new Sound habits into your job, your vacations, and family time—in short, how to master Sound Living.

THE PROCESS

Too many people out there have a basement full of seldom-used fitness equipment, a bookshelf packed with weight-loss and fitness titles, and a closet full of barely worn exercise clothing and shoes. They're all victims of the same problem. Have you ever written a hefty check to a fitness center only to waste your money? Have you ever started to diet, lost some weight, and then gained it all back—and then some? Have you ever stopped eating chocolate or bread or butter in January only to find yourself bingeing in February? Welcome to the club.

Many of my clients are rich, and some of them are famous. But they share the same struggles as anyone else. I've found that it doesn't much matter how much money a person makes or how famous or influential she is—every one of us faces many of the same challenges when it comes to meeting fitness goals. Or, as my mother always says, we all put our trousers on one leg at a time.

Throughout the book, you'll get to know some of my clients who have successfully completed their 6-week Sound Mind, Sound Body program. You will see that the journey for each of them was not an easy one. There were moments when each felt that she couldn't do another repetition or drink another protein shake.

Not unlike Dorothy in the *Wizard of Oz*, traveling down the yellow brick road, you too can be led off course by the demons of self-doubt, stress, boredom, frustration, and impatience. Stay the course. You'll taste it, you'll feel it, you'll see it—your clothes will fit better, you will be calmer, and you'll be more comfortable with your body and in your relationship to food. I've been there; I've fallen off the path and pulled myself back on again. Every time you fall off of the wellness wagon, pick yourself up and remember your promise. Look in the mirror and tell yourself, "I can make a difference; I will feel a difference."

I know many trainers and health experts who will tell you that sticking to a program is all about willpower. They say if you would just try harder, success would be assured. They tell you to wait it out, and soon you'll love the taste of food without salt or love running on a treadmill. If for some reason you don't come to love it, there must be something wrong with you. Inevitably, you lose your self-confidence, the fitness program slips, and the cycle begins again.

Well, I would like to let you in on a secret: There is absolutely nothing wrong with you. You have the willpower, gumption, and initiative to stick with a *wellness* program. You merely need to learn how to direct your inner drive. The process consists of breaking it down into small, doable steps. You will live with a sense of positive energy and reinforcement. The essence of this program is that there is a will and a need to succeed in all of us. My self-awareness program will help you find it, harness it, and utilize it with the greatest efficiency.

There are numerous books, videos, and programs that tell you how to get fit. While you'll find food plans and workout schedules galore, few of them tell you how to enjoy exercise and eating healthfully. And that's the crux. You can force yourself to exercise for a while or to follow a healthful nutrition plan. But it takes a transformation to exercise for the rest of your life. When you enjoy it, exercise comes so naturally that it no longer feels forced. You will naturally feel drawn toward movement. In fact, you'll soon find that you actually miss exercise when you don't do it. Right now, that may seem impossible. But the key is to learn how to turn on your inner drive.

THE PROMISE

I've spent the past 15 years sharing my personal discovery. I've helped people like Ivana Trump, Heidi Klum, Naomi Campbell, James King, and most recently, Linda Evangelista discover the perfect eating and exercise plans for their specific body types. I've helped high-tech executives find the time to fit fitness into their 15-hour workdays. I've shown gourmet restaurant owners how to resist the buttery dishes served at their establishments. I've gone out to eat with clients at some of the most "dangerous" restaurants and enjoyed nutritious, delicious meals.

Like me, many of my clients weren't the picture of health and fit-

ness when they first stepped in the door of the Madison Square Club. Some came in wearing oversized shirts to hide their bodies. They had tried exercise. They had gone on numerous diets. They had lost weight many times, and gained weight just as many. They had seen themselves skinny and seen themselves fat.

But after 6 weeks on my program, they became not just thinner, fitter, more toned, and more taut; they also became healthier. Their minds and bodies were well, or at least were on the path toward wellness. That creates a radiance that many diet and fitness programs simply can't provide.

Don't let me paint too rosy a picture. The path toward wellness is long and, at times, arduous. It is filled with potholes in the guise of fast-food restaurants, stressful jobs, and demanding mates. In addition, we all have demons that, if we allow them, will sabotage our plans and take us off course. The process of recognizing, embracing, and thwarting these personal devils will take you to new heights. I promise to lead you through the maze of choices presented. I can help clear the path toward spiritual, physical, and emotional wellness, but it is important to realize that you, too, have to commit to the process. Remember, I will help you on your way by presenting the exercises, nutrition, and psychological techniques that you need to prepare for your adventure, but the journey is yours to take.

THE CHALLENGE

We all have the inner strength to reach our goals. The challenge is to locate, harness, and use it in a positive, nurturing, and life-enriching way. Once you harness that power, anything is possible. This can be a life-altering program, not just a 6-week diet and exercise plan. It takes commitment, and you must be ready to change. In the following quote, spiritual and political leader Nelson Mandela eloquently expresses some thoughts to keep in mind before embarking on your path. It is my dream that you will be inspired to reach for your greatest potential.

Our deepest fear is not that we are inadequate. Our deepest fear is that we are powerful beyond measure. It is our light, not our darkness, that most frightens us.

We ask ourselves, who am I to be brilliant, gorgeous, talented, and fabulous? Actually, who are you NOT to be?

Your playing small doesn't serve the world. There is nothing enlightened about shrinking so that other people won't feel insecure around you.

We are born to manifest the glory of the spirit that is within us, and as we let our own light shine, we actually unconsciously give other people permission to do the same.

As we are liberated from our own fear, our presence automatically liberates others.

—Nelson Mandela, 1994

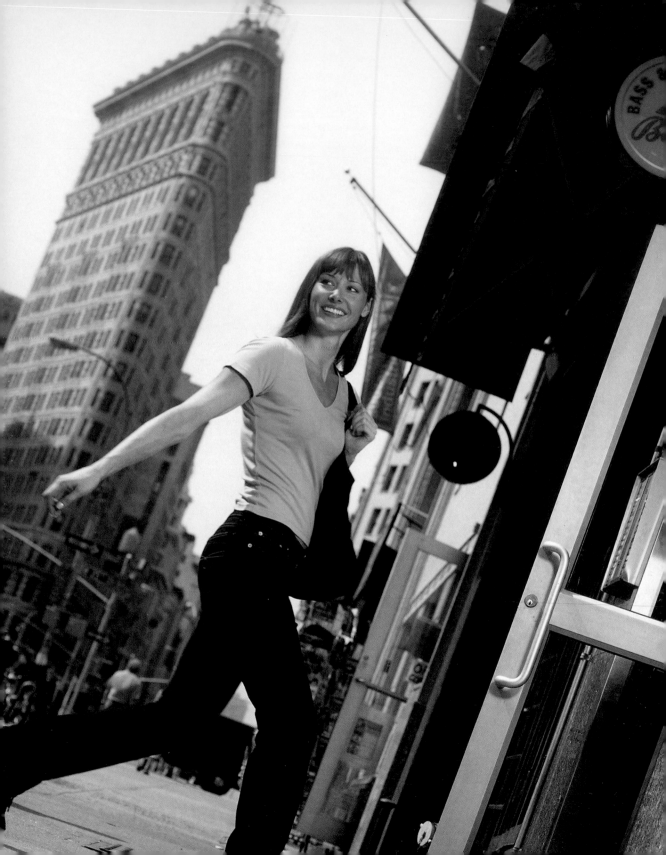

Chapter One

SOUND BEGINNINGS

BEFORE SHE STARTED training with me 2 years ago, Cindy Gallop hated to exercise. She loathed it. "When I lived in the United Kingdom, I used to pay huge amounts of money to feel guilty because I never went to the fitness centers that I joined. Then after I moved to New York and gained some weight, I decided yet again that I needed to start working out. So, I looked for a club with just one thing in mind: proximity to my apartment," she told me.

The Madison Square Club was just 2 blocks from Cindy's apartment. As she had in the past, Cindy signed up for multiple months' worth of training sessions. But unlike the past, this time Cindy actually showed up. In fact, I see Cindy 5 to 7 days a week at 5:30 A.M.

What made the difference? With my help, she found her balance. I helped her integrate fitness and healthy eating habits into her life, for the first time making them things that she actually enjoyed, looked forward to, and felt as if she couldn't live without. It didn't hurt that she carved out a terrific body in the process.

She's not my only client who has experienced a dramatic transformation. "Each of my workout sessions feels like magic," Jeanne Levy-Hinte, another client, told me. "I'm always surprised."

And yet another client, Marcy Engelman, said, "This is the most painless, most effective workout I've ever done. I don't have to deprive myself. It just works. It's a formula that works."

Why are Cindy, Jeanne, Marcy, and hundreds of other clients finding such a strong source of motivation during a time when three out of every five people who start a workout program fall off the wagon? What's the secret? What's the formula?

It's balanced training, with body, mind, and spirit. Through the Sound Mind, Sound Body program, I'm going to show you six easy steps to turn on your inner drive and keep it running. You'll learn how to Soundly combine eating, exercise, and thinking habits into a balanced and joyful program that you can easily stick to for the rest of your life.

You'll take your very first step right now, by carefully planning your future. You see, one of the most important secrets to firing up your inner drive is making sure you start on the right foot.

Many of the choices you make at the beginning of a wellness program, from the goals you set to what gym you join, will affect your internal motivation. Make the right choices now, and you'll eliminate excuses later on.

TAKE A HARD LOOK AT YOUR LIFE

When Michelle Blank came to me, she had been working 10 to 12 hours a day, 7 days a week, as a technical executive. Each morning for 3 years straight, she would wake up, look in the mirror, and tell herself, "I have to do something about this. I'm going to be 'good' today." Then her day would start, and she'd forget about being good.

"As miserable as I was with myself, my head just wasn't ready to make that commitment," she told me later. "I just kept waking up and saying that I was going to do something, but 3 years went by and I was never 'good.'" Over those 3 years, she gained 25 pounds. Her knees and back were starting to ache. Michelle was in her midforties, but she felt like an "old lady." Finally, one day, she looked in the mirror and said to herself, "Who is this person? This person is not me!"

"I knew that if I was going to do this—if I was going to start exercising and losing weight—I would have to give something up," she told me. "I was just too busy. It takes mental energy, focus, and a commitment to be healthy. I had to create that energy and the space to work healthy habits into my life. It was a mind shift."

She couldn't give up her job, so she adjusted her sleep schedule. Michelle started getting up at 4:30 A.M. to ready herself for her 5:45 A.M. appointments with me. The first 3 weeks were difficult. On Saturdays, she would return home after her workout and sleep on her couch for hours. But soon, her new fitness and healthy eating habits transformed her body, mind, and spirit, giving her renewed energy.

Before you start your 6-week journey to wellness, you too must make that mind shift. You must take a hard look at your schedule and find 4 to 5 hours a week for your fitness program. You must take a hard look at your life to make sure your mind is truly in the game. You must make a commitment.

To find time, you could, like Michelle, lose some sleep. But do that only if it's sleep you can afford to lose. Over the next 6 weeks, I guarantee that your new healthy habits will infuse your body with energy and vigor you didn't know you could have. But these new energizing habits won't make up for consistent sleep loss. Everyone's sleep needs are slightly different. But if you feel the urge to take naps in the middle of the day—especially 3 weeks into your program—you're not getting enough sleep. Here are some tips to help you find time for your new lifestyle.

Block out time for yourself. Don't feel guilty about it. I use a computerized calendar and, well in advance, block out an hour each day to exercise or even to just spend time alone. For my exercise time, I try to limit the sessions in my club so I can use the equipment without distraction. Get rid of your pager, cell phone, and other communication devices. Turn them off, unplug from the world, and block out 30 to 60 minutes a day as your personal time to be away from everyone.

Be firm. I learned this the hard way. I run a business with more than 300 clients a week. If I tried to please everyone all the time, I would burn out. So I've learned to delegate, to call people back when *I'm* ready, and to gracefully and firmly say no. Remember: You're much better for yourself and everyone in your life when you are rested and focused.

Make tough decisions. I once heard a pastor say, "You show me your date book and your checkbook register, and I'll tell you where your priorities are." He had a point. What you spend your money on and where you spend your time and energy should be things you feel are important. If they're not, your life is out of balance. For a few days, keep track of your hours by writing everything into your time planner, including TV time and social time. Where do you spend your time? Did you need to spend 12 hours a day at work? How much time do you spend watching television? How much time do you spend talking to coworkers?

Confront your energy robbers. People can either give energy or take it. If you surround yourself with people who drain you of energy, you'll always feel tired. Make a mental note of how others around you make you feel. Are your spouse, friends, and family constantly leaning on you for emotional support? Maybe it's time to take a step back. Are you in a tumultuous relationship? Maybe that person is not the right person for you. If this sounds too difficult right now, rest assured, I'll tell you everything you need to know about creating more inner energy in chapter 5.

MAKE A COMMITMENT

You must not only create time for your new habits but also firmly commit yourself to the process. As Michelle now likes to say, "This is a lifestyle change. If I can do it, anyone can. You need to be there mentally. You don't just change your habits for 6 weeks, you change them for the rest of your life."

You are about to embark on an incredible 6-week journey to wellness. During that journey, I will show you the best path to take and help clear debris out of your way. But you will also need to participate. I can show you the way, but I can't carry you. You must do the walking. And sometimes, you'll be walking uphill.

You're not the only one making a commitment. I am, too. I promise to be

Contract for a Fitness Transformation

I, _____(Your name), promise to strive to the best of my ability to follow David's Sound Mind, Sound Body approach to wellness. When I slip up, even though I've tried my hardest, I will not feel guilty because I will have tried my hardest. Instead, I'll just pick myself back up and continue the program with renewed zeal. _____ (Your signature)

I, David Kirsch, promise to give you the tools you need to make Sound eating choices, follow a Sound fitness routine, and create a Sound Mind. When you are facing your inner demons, I promise to be at your side, giving you the advice you need to continue down your path to wellness.

_____

with you every step of the way, just as I am with my clients. When I start new clients at my club, I call them often, just to check in. As Stephanie Fray, one of my clients, told me, "You are so good at gauging my moods and mindset. You seem to be able to sense when I need extra support. Last night I was about to eat a chocolate-chip cookie when the phone rang. It was you."

I've worked with so many clients for so many years that I know where the natural stumbling blocks are and when you will encounter them on your road to wellness. I promise that throughout this book I will point out those stumbling blocks and help you surmount them. You can safely navigate any rough spot as long as you are firmly committed from the start. You can strengthen that commitment by signing the "Contract for a Fitness Transformation."

ACCEPT YOUR LIMITS

Aristotle once recommended all things in moderation, so why do so many people continue to overeat and overexercise? Back in the 1970s, a lot of trainers used the phrase "no pain, no gain" to describe exercise. The belief was that you had to put your body through a certain amount of discomfort in order to see any results.

Most trainers now know that's a bunch of hogwash. That thinking has

derailed more than one fitness program, and it's the kind of thinking that you must banish from your brain before you take the next step in your wellness journey.

My client Jeanne learned this the hard way before she met me. She was an obsessive exerciser. She could run for 3 or more hours at a time, and she enjoyed it. But the obsession took a toll on her body, and she suffered everything from back pain to frozen shoulders to hamstring pulls. She would work out obsessively for a week, then spend the next week recuperating in bed. When she began training with me, one of the first areas we focused on was for her to find a way to push herself "just right," rather than overdoing it. Now she's toned, fit, and injury-free.

Whether you have past injuries, like Jeanne, or like some of my other clients, you have a chronic illness, you must accept your body for what it will offer you on any given day. You don't have to forgo exercise because of a health condition, but you should modify your program accordingly. Always listen to your body. Pain has no place in an exercise routine.

So promise me this right now: You will not make fitness a competition to see how much you can put your body through. Neither will you see how many excuses you can come up with to blow off your routine. You will listen to your body and give it what it needs. You'll learn more about how to do this in the following chapters. Also, before starting your program, I want you to do two things:

1. Talk to your doctor about your plans. Some diseases and health conditions will complicate your fitness routine. For example, if you have diabetes, you may need to pay careful attention to your blood sugar during exercise.

2. If you are going to work with a trainer, make sure the trainer is knowledgeable about any health conditions you have. I have a client who needs to carry a fruit shake around during his exercise routine to prevent his blood sugar from dropping too low. I understand his needs; not all trainers do.

FIND YOUR MOTIVATION

Many people think motivation is a genetic trait, that some people have it and others don't. That's simply not true. Yes, some people do have more drive than others. Also, exercise comes more naturally to some, especially those with bodies naturally suited to athletics. But motivation really isn't about drive. It's about Sound Training.

If you slog through the same boring workout day after day, your motivation will sag. *My* motivation would plummet if I did the same exercises day in and day out. The most important element in a successful fit-

ness program is variety. Keep it fresh. Make every session different, and your motivation will stay strong. In my Sound Training program, I'll show you how to do just that.

Motivation is also about confidence. Research shows that self-esteem plays a huge role in adherence to any new habit, whether that habit is flossing your teeth, eating less fat, or lifting weights. If you believe you can do it, you will do it. If you don't think you can, you won't. I'll teach you more about how to improve your confidence in chapter 5.

Motivation is also about setting clear, realistic goals and seeing regular results. You may say, "I want to get fit and lose weight." But that isn't a specific enough target. Instead, break that goal down into mini goals, so that you see improvement every week. I'll show you how to do that in chapter 2.

Finally, motivation is about support. Some people can find that support easily among their family and friends. Others need a little extra help, and that's why they turn to personal trainers.

I once overheard a conversation between two of my clients in the gym. One said to the other, "So many of my friends ask me why I still need a trainer after so many years of working out. If this were only a matter of lifting weights and knowing the right exercises to do, they would be right. I could do this on my own. But it's about more than that. It's about pushing myself past where I normally would go. I need a trainer to give me that extra push."

A trainer can help you to stick to your program. A trainer will keep you honest. If you feel like blowing off a session, you actually have to call your trainer to cancel. You'll be disap-pointing two people rather than just one. And your best excuses don't sound so convincing when you have to say them out loud to someone else.

But you must hire the *right* trainer for this to work (see "Choosing the Right Trainer").

Choosing the Right Trainer

Here are some questions to ask yourself to make sure your trainer is right for you:

1. Can you trust him? I work with a lot of trainers, and I always use this simple test to see if they have the confidence it takes to train me: I look them in the eye. If they can't return that eye contact, then I know I'm not going to feel comfortable with them spotting me or directing my routine.

2. Do you like him? This may seem like a silly question, but it's an important one. You want a trainer whom you enjoy being around. Otherwise, you'll be more likely to cancel your ap-pointments.

3. Does the trainer motivate you in a positive way? You want someone who empowers you to believe in yourself and your abilities, not someone who scares you or makes you feel inade-quate.

4. Does the trainer have the right credentials? Make sure the trainer is certified through one of two organizations: the American Council on Exercise (ACE) or the American College of Sports Medicine (ACSM).

5. When the trainer describes your program, is it one that you feel motivated to complete? If not, is the trainer willing to modify the program to meet your individual needs and interests?

6. Does the trainer understand your goals and support them?

7. Has the trainer asked you about you?

8. If you have any health concerns, is the trainer knowledgeable enough to deal with those is-sues? Some trainers are specifically knowledgeable about special needs such as osteo-porosis or osteoarthritis.

9. Has the trainer tested your strength, flexibility, and cardiovascular endurance before de-signing your program?

I've heard too many stories from my clients about negative experiences with personal trainers. They worked with trainers who pushed them too hard, getting them injured. Or they worked with trainers who designed boring routines. They worked with trainers who didn't listen to their needs, who didn't stay involved enough during the workout, and who simply didn't care about their results.

I'm not saying I'm the only good trainer out there. There are lots of good ones. There are lots of great ones, and you'll be able to find one in your area. But you should put as much homework into hiring a trainer as you do when purchasing a car. Shop around. Don't hire the first person you meet.

WHERE TO EXERCISE

Where you choose to exercise plays a huge role in whether you continue to exercise. It's one of the most important decisions you'll make.

Many people immediately think that they'll be better off in a commercial gym setting where they can move from machine to machine, take guided classes, and consult with on-staff trainers. But commercial gyms aren't for everyone. First and most important, exercising at a gym involves exercising with and in front of other people. This can feel intimidating to

you, especially if you don't feel confident using the equipment or if you feel embarrassed about the shape or size of your body. It also means that you may have to wait to use equipment, and occasionally have to deal with other people's bad gym etiquette.

I'm not saying that you should never exercise at a commercial gym. For some people, working out at a fitness club is inspiring. For others, it's not. Decide which type of person you are before making a commitment either way. Your honest answers to the following questions will help you decide whether to exercise at home or at a club:

◆ Would you skip a workout because you didn't feel like getting in your car and driving to the gym?
◆ Are finances a concern?
◆ Are you comfortable exercising with other people?
◆ How do you feel about crowds?
◆ Do you prefer to keep to yourself, avoiding small talk with strangers?
◆ How flexible is your schedule? To exercise consistently, do you need to exercise very early in the morning or very late at night?

Evaluate your answers and determine if you're more likely to be successful with a home gym or a fitness club. If you've chosen to go with a commercial gym, read on. If you've decided to create a gym at home, skip to "Building Your Home Exercise Oasis" on page 10.

CHOOSING A COMMERCIAL GYM

If you've decided that a commercial gym will motivate you best, your next step is finding the right gym for you. By doing your homework, visiting numerous clubs, and taking the following characteristics into consideration, you can find the gym that best suits your needs.

Your age. It's been my experience that older, less experienced clients tend to feel more comfortable in more private, discreet settings. The smaller the club, the less likely you'll feel as if you're in a pickup joint. Stay away from the "meat market clubs" if you want to avoid being gawked at or chatted up during your workouts.

Your fitness background. There are different types of clubs—bodybuilding gyms (with lots of intimidating equipment and people), women-friendly gyms that feature more classes (such as aerobics and Spinning), fitness malls (mega-gyms that try to offer you everything and span entire city blocks), and smaller, more intimate clubs. Pick a club that best matches your fitness background and interests. It's very helpful to exer-

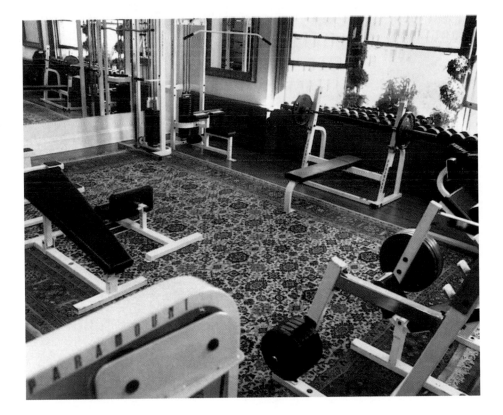

cise in an environment with like-minded people, so the people at the gym, from the trainers to the other members, should complement your fitness goals.

Your past excuses. Make a list of all the reasons you don't exercise or have stopped exercising in the past. This list will help you focus on the things to avoid in your new health club. I found this process very helpful when I conceptualized and built the Madison Square Club. I thought about all the reasons people either don't go to a health club, or, if they sign up, don't continue to attend regularly. I used this approach to create an environment that addressed my particular clients' needs. I built a *club* with oriental rugs, natural light, and flowers—not a *gym*.

Your financial constraints. Two hundred dollars can buy you an annual membership or merely 1 month's dues. What amenities are you looking for? Do you want a full-service juice bar, personal training, and more? These things cost money and will bump up the cost of your membership.

BUILDING YOUR HOME EXERCISE OASIS

The first tool you'll need is a private exercise sanctum. My dad's basement gym would most likely inspire only my dad, who is one of the rare few who naturally love working out. But it offered one of the most important elements of motivation—the fitness "refuge." Now, Dad's private sanctum was a cross between a medieval torture chamber and a principal's office, but it was his!

Some of my fondest memories of my father involve spending time with him in this sparsely decorated yet incredibly overcrowded space. You would need a compass to navigate the maze of equipment in this 10- by 15-foot rectangle of unfinished basement. It was chilly in the winter and hot, damp, and airless during the summer. There were no windows, yet I loved being there. When we were downstairs, everyone, even my mother, knew not to disturb us.

Dad taught me the importance of creating an escape space, a temple, a safety zone. We all need a place where we feel safe, protected, and nurtured.

Whether your space is big or small, plain or deluxe, filled with lots of equipment or none at all (see "Outfitting Your Home Gym"), the most important ingredient is that it conveys a sense of well-being. It must invite you in and envelope you in your own sense of peace and calm.

Your home gym can become the perfect oasis or a complete waste of space, depending on how you set it up. First, find the location in your home that you think is the most conducive to exercise. It should be a place you can call your own, one that is off-limits to anyone who might interrupt. Here are some pointers to follow in creating your own exercise haven.

Outfitting Your Home Gym

To do my Sound Training program right, you'll need the following:

◆ **An exercise mat.** You need a mat for stretching, floor work, and abdominal exercises.

◆ **A sturdy, adjustable bench.** Buy a bench that can be set at both an incline and a decline position. This bench is your most important investment, so be willing to spend a few hundred dollars for a high-quality commercial bench. It'll last you 10 to 12 years (or longer) if you take good care of it. Stay away from benches with bar racks and leg curl attachments. You don't need them; they're cumbersome and they get in the way. Lie on the bench at the store and make sure it feels both sturdy and comfortable. Benches come in different widths; I prefer the wider ones.

◆ **A set of dumbbells.** Start with dumbbells ranging from 3 to 15 pounds. You may buy heavier dumbbells as you get stronger, but this range will be enough for beginners. Look for smaller dumbbells, which are less clumsy to lift. Pick them up and handle them in the store to make sure they feel comfortable to hold.

◆ **A pair of ankle weights.** Start with 5 pounds and increase from there. If you are feeling ambitious and can afford it, purchase a second pair of 10-pound ankle weights. The 10-pound pair is probably going to be the heaviest you will use and will give your legs a major workout for a long time.

◆ **A chinup bar or squat rack.** I prefer squat racks because you can use them for squats, hanging knee raises, and other exercises as well as chinups. Also, some homes are not equipped with sturdy enough doorways to accommodate chinup bars. If yours does, however, the chinup bar is all you'll need.

◆ **A water bottle.** You need to stay plenty hydrated during exercise, so keep a filled water bottle nearby. Or, you can go upscale and invest in a water cooler.

◆ **An optional medicine ball and large exercise ball.** You can find both of these at large sporting-goods stores. They will come in handy for abdominal and leg work.

◆ **A stereo.** When he was younger, my dad didn't believe in having music in the gym. He has since given in, and now regularly plays Frank Sinatra, Ella Fitzgerald, and Miles Davis. Whether you listen to rock, classic '70s (my favorite), or classical, your music should make you feel inspired to work out.

Keep it light. If you don't have access to natural light, use generous amounts of overhead lighting. Lots of good light is energizing.

Make the space reflect who you are and what you need. I fill my gym with fresh flowers, beautiful photographs, and great books and magazines. It is my refuge, my safe haven from all that hounds me throughout the day. My dad's gym included a vast library of bodybuilding magazines dating back to the early 1960s. However you choose to decorate it, make it uniquely yours.

Use mirrors. Even Dad's home gym included a small mirror that we could use to check our form as we exercised. Additionally, a few mirrors can convert a small space into one that seems much larger. I've designed gyms in tiny rooms that ultimately looked quite spacious with the help of a few well-placed mirrors.

Keep the space as open and clutter-free as possible. Stick to the basics. Don't fall victim to every new toy that appears on a television infomercial. Too much clutter is distracting and potentially dangerous. Donate the ab rollers and other unused exercise equipment, get a receipt, and use it as a tax deduction. Make your redesigned home gym pay for itself.

My dad has come a long way since the early basement days. He and Mom now live in a house where Dad has claimed a beautiful finished and carpeted basement with mirrors and pictures of all the bodybuilding greats—Steve Reeves, John Grimek, Arnold Schwarzenegger. He has kept all of his old equipment and added some modern pieces, such as a Paramount cable machine. In spite of the modern feel, it's still as cramped as always, just the way he likes it.

A FRESH START

Now you're almost ready for step two of the 6-week program: goal setting. Before you move on, however, I have a little homework assignment for you. You'll feel more motivated throughout the program if you make a fresh start. So, before you take your next step, do the following:

1. Purchase new exercise clothes.

2. Purchase new exercise shoes.

3. Create an exercise space, overhaul your current home gym, or join a commercial gym.

4. I'll go into more detail about Sound Eating in chapter 4, but to get started now, raid your kitchen cabinets and refrigerator for the following items and toss them in the trash:
◆ Foods made from white flour, including bread and pasta
◆ Foods composed mainly of empty sugars, including candy and soda

◆ Highly processed foods, including potato chips (even the nonfat ones), rice, rice cakes, crackers, and just about anything else that comes in a box, bag, or can
◆ Anything with artificial sweeteners, including diet sodas and diet frozen foods

5. Hit the grocery and health food stores. Use this list:
◆ Fresh vegetables, especially spinach, kale, broccoli, beans, and sweet potatoes
◆ Fresh fruits, especially berries
◆ Organic sirloin or buffalo
◆ Organic ground turkey breast
◆ Fresh fish
◆ Pasta made from a nonwheat whole grain such as spelt
◆ Olive oil
◆ Raw sugar
◆ Whey protein powder
◆ Whole grain bread
◆ Eggs
◆ Yogurt
◆ Frozen yogurt
◆ Raw nuts
◆ Protein bars

6. Buy a new notebook or three-ring binder. This is a good place to write down your answers to the Sound Thinking exercises in chapter 5. You can also use it to record your thoughts and feelings throughout the program.

7. Pick a date more than 6 weeks in the future to celebrate the new you. You might celebrate by taking a 4-day weekend at an exotic location or by having a bunch of friends over for a "boot camp." (I'll tell you everything you need to know about boot camps in chapter 6.)

8. Spend some time alone and think back to all of your failed fitness and nutrition plans. What went wrong? What was the deciding excuse that you used to stop your new habit? Once you list all of your past excuses, brainstorm ways that *you* can ensure that they won't crop up again.

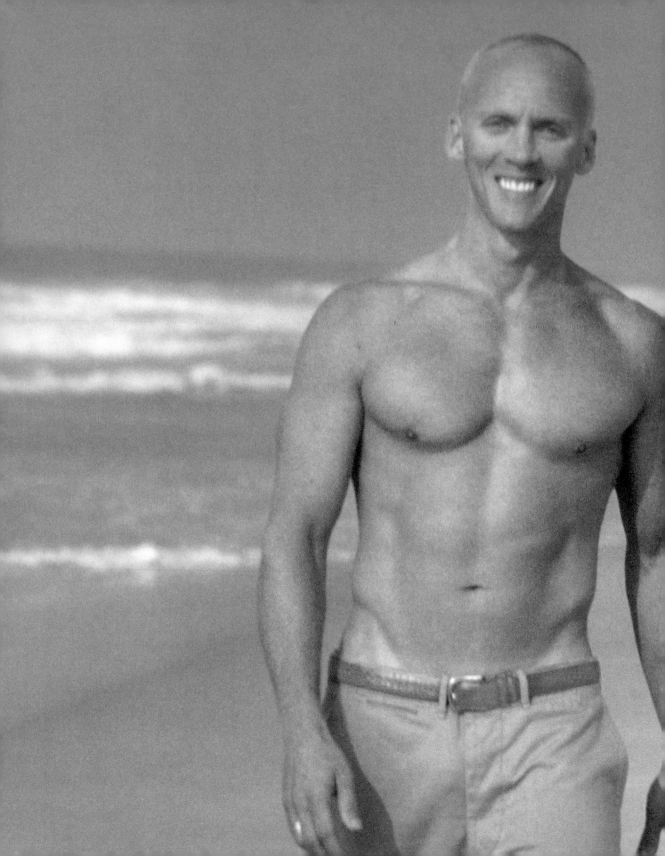

Chapter Two

SOUND CONFIDENCE

PEOPLE SOMETIMES sabotage themselves from the very beginning by setting impossible goals. For example, when a client tells me she wants to look like someone else, such as a famous actress, a red flag goes up for me. I wonder why this person would want to look like someone else. Why doesn't she like herself? Will she ever be satisfied with her physical appearance?

"There's plenty wrong with me," a client might tell me. Sure, maybe he needs to lose a few pounds, tighten up around the middle, or build more defined muscles. But that doesn't mean there is anything intrinsically wrong with his natural body.

Actually, life would be a pretty tedious visual existence if every woman looked like Jennifer Aniston and every guy looked like Brad Pitt. Variety is what makes us interesting. Homogeneity is boring. You are unique!

Your ultimate goal is to look and feel the best you can, not to look like some beauty queen, model, actor, or actress. Your best body begins with and builds on your natural body. Don't use magazines, books, or even your neighbor as your measuring stick. Instead, set realistic goals and celebrate the many personal achievements you make during your journey. Each step you take is a cause for celebration.

For step two in your Sound Mind, Sound Body program, I'm going to show you how to break six large, important goals down into small, man-

Sound Results

After spending 6 weeks with me and my Sound Mind, Sound Body program, you will develop a better sense of self, sharper mental acuity, and an overall feeling of wellness. Upon completion of the program, you will:

◆ Feel better about yourself

◆ Feel better about the people in your life

◆ Feel better about how the people in your life feel about you

◆ Feel and act more assertive and self-assured

◆ Look at food in a different way—not as an escape or a punishment, but as your positive reward

◆ Look at exercise in a different way—not as punishment or torture, but as fun and nurturing

I'm so confident about these results that I'll even give you a way to test how well the program worked for you. Take the following test today, and then again in 6 weeks. After you complete the 6-week program, you will be pleasantly surprised at the changes in your answers.

1. How do you see yourself physically? How do you believe other people perceive you physically? How do other people say they perceive you physically?

2. What are your goals for this program? Do you want to look slimmer? Do you want to be stronger and look more toned?

3. What is your attitude toward food? Are you using food to cover your emotions? Do you feel imprisoned by your cravings?

4. What is your attitude toward exercise? Does it feel like a chore?

5. What is your attitude toward life? What hand of cards do you feel have you been dealt? Have people treated you unfairly?

I guarantee that if you adhere to the basic tenets of my program, you will feel better, perceive yourself and others in a better light, and have an overall improved sense of self. Oh—and you'll look fantastic.

ageable chunks to build your confidence and keep you motivated throughout the program.

GOAL #1:
CREATING YOUR BEST BODY

This is the goal that probably influenced you to buy this book: your body. So what is a good body? The ideal is different for men and women.

WAIST-TO-HIP RATIO (FOR WOMEN)

It's an ancient truism that one of the most attractive features a woman can possess is a slim waist and proportionately wider hips. Not only does this drive men wild, but also it's good for your health. If you're the type of woman who gains weight in your abdomen, you're at greater risk for heart disease than someone who tends to gain weight in the butt and thighs. So use that as an important motivator to slim down.

To gauge your progress, measure the circumference of your waist and the circumference of your hips once a week. Then divide your waist measurement by your hip measurement to calculate your waist-to-hip ratio. For optimal health, you want a ratio under 0.8.

CHEST-TO-WAIST RATIO (FOR MEN)

One of the most attractive features a man can possess is an upper body shaped like an upside-down triangle. The base of the triangle is the chest and shoulders, and the tip is the abdomen. Besides looking great, a good chest-to-waist ratio lessens the risk of heart disease and other health problems. So use that as an important motivator to slim down. To gauge your progress, measure the circumference of your chest and the circumference of your waist once a week. Then subtract your waist measurement from your chest measurement. Ten is a good goal.

THE FIVE BASIC BODY TYPES

To set motivating and realistic goals for slimming down and shaping up, you must first consider your body type. My Sound Training plan is designed to help you to deal best with the body type you were born with, accentuating the positive and minimizing the negative. (See page 116 for more on body types.)

The apple. Many women will recognize this body type. You're an apple if you carry most of your body weight in your belly, hips, and rear end but have relatively thin legs.

Many apple types have learned that an oversize sweater paired with jeans or tights will accent their slim legs and hide their middles. This ability to hide belly bulge with clothing can decrease motivation to change their body shapes. But apples truly have more at stake than the other body types. Because apples carry most of their body fat near their hearts, they are at an increased risk for heart disease. Use that fear—and that waist-to-hip or chest-to-waist ratio that you measured—as your inspiration to get moving.

The pear. This is a common body type for women. You're a pear if you carry most of your body weight in your hips, butt, and thighs but have a fairly flat belly.

Unlike apples, pears are usually extremely motivated to slim down. It's much harder to hide your thighs and butt in a swimsuit, a pair of jeans, and most other types of clothing than it is to hide your belly.

The stick. I usually see this body type in men who, despite their best efforts, can't seem to build any muscle. You're a stick if you've ever had sand kicked on you at the beach, especially if it was your girlfriend kicking the sand!

Scientists call this body type the ectomorph. You have naturally small bones, which will make it difficult to build overall heft. Concentrate on building a solid chest and firm arms and abs instead of building thickness. Core foundation exercises plus good nutrition with lots of lean protein will help you achieve your goals.

The round type. Not to be confused with the apple, the round body type is a symmetrical person who is overweight and/or large framed. Also called the endomorph by scientists, this body type is genetically predisposed to roundness. When you are heavy all over with no defining body shape—you're not top heavy or bottom heavy—you fall into the round category.

The symmetrically fit type. If you've been exercising for a while and are at your goal weight but are looking for the extra edge in toning, then you fall into this body type. Also called a mesomorph by scientists, you have an average bone structure, neither overly large nor small. Every once in a while, a part of your body might bug you. One month it's your abs, the next it's your butt, but overall, your body type is symmetrical. This is the easiest body type to whip into shape.

My program will help you whittle that abdominal fat if you're an apple, thin those thighs if you're a pear, build up your musculature if you're a stick, slim down all over if you're round, and generally firm up if you're symmetrically fit. It's a fact, though, that your body shape will not change overnight, and that's why, regardless of your body type, you need incremental goals to keep yourself motivated.

	Week 1	Week 2	Week 3	Week 4	Week 5	Week 6
Waist-to-hip ratio (Women) (waist measurement ÷ hip measurement)						
Chest-to-waist ratio (Men) (chest measurement-waist measurement)						
HDL level	–	–	–	–		
LDL level	–	–	–	–		
Resting heart rate (count beats for 30 seconds and multiply by 2)						
Overall well-being (1–10)						

GOAL #2:
DEVELOPING WELLNESS AND WELL-BEING

Many people focus solely on physical appearance when setting goals, but how your body looks is just one aspect of the big picture. Most of us assume that looking better will help us feel better. In some cases, that's true, but not for the reasons that you may think. The exercise and eating habits you adopt to carve the body you desire will do more than help you look your best; they will boost your mood, burn off stress, and boost your overall well-being.

Isn't that really what's at stake? If you have a killer body but feel miserable all the time, what good is it? Looking good comes from the inside.

By changing some of the circumstances in your life (being sedentary, feeling stressed, staying in a bad relationship), you can remove the encumbrances that are preventing you from looking and feeling your best.

That's why your first goal is improving your overall internal health, your happiness and wellness. Before you start your 6-week program, gather and write down as many of the following variables as possible in your notebook. The sample chart above should get you started.

HDL AND LDL CHOLESTEROL LEVELS
Your blood cholesterol levels provide important information about your health status. They also serve as a

good indicator that your healthy diet and exercise program is working. But don't focus on your total number. Your high-density lipoprotein (HDL) cholesterol is your "healthy" cholesterol reading. HDL is the type of blood fat that escorts other fats out of your arteries. Low-density lipoprotein

From Tight Fit to Right Fit

A lot of people turn to the scale for motivation. I don't believe in weight as a motivator for a number of reasons: Muscle weighs more than fat; it also takes up much less body space. So as you shape up, your weight may not change that dramatically on the scale, even though you are looking much better. Many of my clients have told me that they look like they've lost more weight than the scale indicates. A number of factors affect what you weigh on a particular day, including the food in your belly, the time of the month, and the time of day. The scale simply is not a reliable indicator of your progress.

Some people may not actually need to lose weight as much as they need to redistribute it. For example, some pear-shaped women look as if their thighs are big simply because their arms are so darn skinny. They don't need to lose weight on the scale, but they do need to fill out their shoulders and slim down their thighs.

So if not the scale, what can you use to measure your progress? Your clothing. As you re-shape your body, the fit of your clothes will change. They might look terrible on you! My clients have experienced renewed motivation as they had their "fat" clothes tailored to fit their newly slimmed bodies and as they shopped for smaller clothing sizes.

Think about what's hanging in your closet right now. What fits and what doesn't? Everyone has clothes that used to fit and look great and now no longer do. Put those clothes together in one section. Now put your fat clothes in the front of your closet. These are the clothes that you bought to fit your body as it grew. Put your fat clothes in order from the roomiest to the least roomy. As you follow the program, I want you to work your way down the closet. Here are some incremental goals to look forward to. Get ready to celebrate reaching each and every one of them!

◆ When all of your fat clothes become roomy

◆ When your old jeans fit after you stretch them out

◆ When those same jeans fit right out of the dryer

◆ When your "used to fit" clothes become your fat clothes

◆ When you run out of clothes and must have them tailored or shop for new, smaller outfits

(LDL) cholesterol, however, is the type of blood fat that adheres to your artery walls, setting the stage for heart disease. You want to raise your HDL and lower your LDL. Have your cholesterol levels checked now, and again in 6 weeks.

RESTING HEART RATE

The more fit you become, the lower your heart rate will be. The lower your heart rate, the better you feel and the longer you live. Measure your resting heart rate once a week before you get out of bed in the morning by placing two fingertips on the carotid artery on the side of your neck, counting the beats for 30 seconds, and then multiplying that number by 2. An average resting heart rate for a man is 70 beats per minute; for a woman, it's 75 beats per minute.

OVERALL WELL-BEING

Well-being goes well beyond heart rate and other health indicators. It includes your energy levels , your mental outlook, and even the bounce in your step. Much of this is hard to measure. But one thing is certain: The better your well-being, the better your motivation. And the better your motivation, the better your well-being.

Each week, rate your overall well-being on a scale of 1 to 10, with 1 meaning on the verge of hospitalization and 10 meaning you feel as if you could conquer the world.

GOAL #3:
CONNECTING BODY AND MIND

Your mind is one of the most important "muscles" to hone, train, and improve, but few people think about that when they start a fitness or weight-loss program. I often tell people that their brains need a jump start. In my program, I put a heavy emphasis on using your mind to direct your body. I don't believe in a fixed number of sets or reps. You instinctively know how many repetitions to lift and how many sets to complete. I can teach you how to access that instinct.

Your mind-body connection—key to success of your Sound Mind, Sound Body program—can be thrown off by many factors, from bad nutrition to a poor or nonexistent exercise routine to self-sabotaging behavioral and attitudinal problems. As you progress further along your Sound Mind, Sound Body journey, you'll find that you experience better clarity as your mind-body connection strengthens.

Most kids are completely in touch with their mind-body connections. They know when they have energy to run around and when they don't. They sleep when they're tired and eat when they're hungry. But most of us were strapped into high-chairs and cribs when we were kids, forced to keep regular eating and sleeping schedules, and slowly but surely our natural mind-body connections eroded.

It will take some work for you to get back in touch, but you will. The most important concept for you to master is the maximum perceived rate of exertion, or MPRE. This is your personal guide to how much stress your body can handle. Your MPRE tells you on a scale of 1 to 10 how hard an effort feels. It tells you before you jump into a pool if you'll be able to swim 50 laps or 20. It tells you if you'll be able to safely lift 15 pounds or 20. It tells you when to stop eating, when to take a nap, and when to walk away from a stressful situation.

MPRE is individual to each person. One person's maximum may feel like cake to another. Your MPRE also can change from day to day and hour to hour. What you were able to bench-press on Monday may not be the same on Wednesday. You'll learn more about your MPRE as the program goes along. In the first week, you may at times overdo it or underdo it as you are trying to figure out how hard to push yourself.

As you progress through the program, you can tap into your MPRE using some of the following questions.

1. Is your brain awake as you exercise? Can you feel the muscle being worked? Can you visualize the burn?

2. Are you mindful when you eat, tasting the food, paying attention to your feelings of fullness—or are you unconsciously eating?

3. Have you stopped counting the number of times you lift a weight, and instead are you focusing on muscle exhaustion?

4. Have you altered an exercise because you felt it would be more effective?

5. Did you go to sleep earlier because you felt you needed the extra rest?

6. Did you end a negative and potentially harmful relationship because it no longer gave you the sense of support and strength that you needed?

GOAL #4:
FINDING YOUR STRENGTH

When many people start fitness programs, they know intuitively that they will get stronger, but few of them realize how much these strength goals can motivate them onward. Every move up to a new dumbbell weight is a major accomplishment. Throughout your 6-week program, focus on two specific exercises, writing down your "before" results right now, and then writing in how you do on this test once a week.

Pushup. This tests your upper-body strength, including your chest, shoulders, and arms. Either use the standard pushup position on the balls of your feet or, if you lack the chest strength to do a Standard Pushup, start on your knees. But the form is the same (see page 45). Then try them on the balls of your feet and consider that your strength victory for the week. Your chest must come within a fist's distance of the ground. (If you think you'll cheat, put a small apple on the floor under your chest and make sure your chest touches the apple each time.) Make sure you push all the way up with your back flat. Note how many you can do without resting.

If you can't do one pushup with good form from the balls of your feet, do them first with your knees on the ground.

Crunch. This tests your abdominal muscle strength and endurance. Lie on a mat with your feet flat on the floor and your knees bent at a 90-degree angle (see page 101). Go at a pace of one crunch every 3 seconds, or 20 a minute. How many can you do with good form?

GOAL #5:

MASTERING YOUR EATING HABITS

Sound Eating is all about making sound choices. It's not about deprivation. You'll learn more about how to make those sound choices when you take the next step in your journey. For now, however, set some goals to help you keep your nutritional habits on track.

Sound Mind, Sound Body Success Story

When I first started training, I told David that I wanted to improve my overall fitness. He looked me up and down and then said, "Okay, let's start by lifting your butt."

I soon moved from my butt to my abs. Each time I achieved a goal, I moved on to the next. Each goal was reasonable and attainable. The consistent results motivated me to get back to the club so I could advance to the next step.

I had always exercised, but this goal-setting method helped me to become committed to training three times a week. I now understand that fitness isn't an absolute, all-or-nothing proposition. It's a process that you build on layer by layer. You get a little better in one area and you build up a little more to the next. You keep building up and building up.

—Desiree Gruber

Too often, people see eating as an all-or-nothing endeavor. They ban their most craved foods from their diets and then berate themselves when they slip up and gobble down that chocolate kiss or french fry. This only leads to further bingeing, and soon their healthy eating habits are a thing of the past.

That's where goal setting comes in. If you see your eating habits as a journey with easily attainable baby steps, you'll be much less likely to completely fall off the wagon any time you feel you've slipped up. Instead, you'll simply pick yourself back up with renewed zeal.

Here are some Sound Eating questions worth asking yourself.

1. When you sit down to eat, do you realize that you have a choice?

2. When you sit down to eat, do you reassess your food choice and change your selection from a hamburger to a grilled chicken sandwich?

3. When you sit down to eat, do you taste your food and enjoy the experience?

4. When you sit down to eat, are you relaxed, unstressed, and conscious of your meal?

5. When you find yourself reaching for a food that tends to make you feel guilty, do you pause and reflect about what's causing you to reach for this food?

6. When you eat something that you wish you hadn't, do you shrug off the guilt and resolve to do better next time?

Now that you've taken an inventory of where you are and laid out a map with bite-size goals for where you're going, you're ready to investigate the next step in the journey to wellness.

GOAL #6:
DEVELOPING YOUR MENTAL FITNESS

I don't train minds as much as I train people to use their minds more fully—to focus on engaging their brains, if you will. Removing obstacles from your path is one of my chief job functions as your coach, and it will help you take a relatively smooth trip on the road to wellness.

To push your body toward its potential, your mind must be strong. If you lack self-esteem, you won't believe that you can do that extra pushup. If you let people walk all over you, you'll skip your workout every time someone asks you to do something for them. If you have a short fuse and a lot of negative energy, you won't possess the strength you need to move forward.

Improving your mental fitness will make you a happier person. Negative emotions—whether you're angry at a coworker, stressed about an upcoming deadline, or depressed about getting passed over for a promotion—can do more than siphon your energy. They can actually destroy your health. Numerous studies show that people who don't feel in control of their lives tend to die sooner from various diseases than people who feel content with the direction of their lives.

It's difficult to see your progress in mental fitness clearly because most of us tend to focus on our mental slipups. To help you see that you really are making progress, each week rate your happiness quotient on a scale of 1 to 10 (1 being completely down in the dumps and 10 feeling heavenly euphoric).

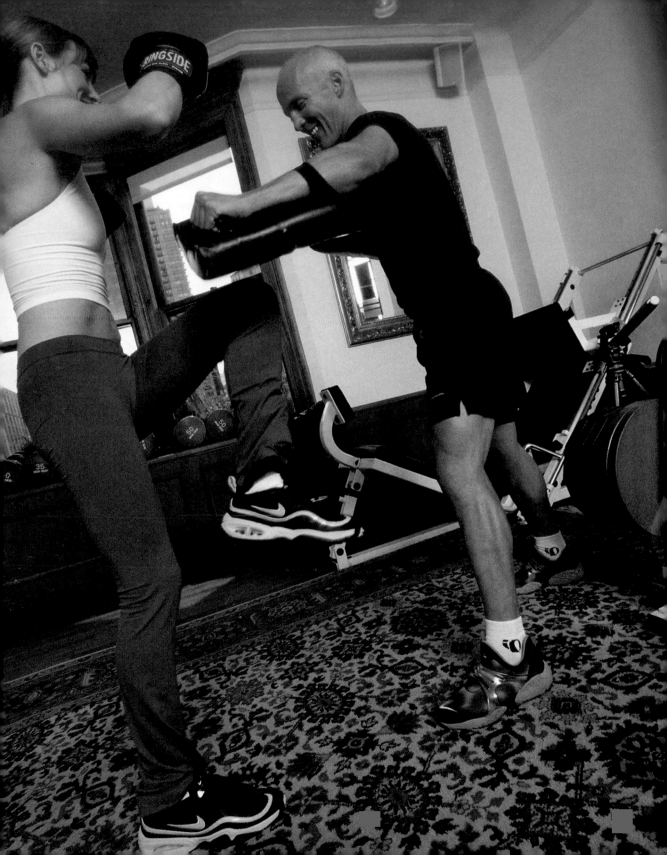

Chapter Three

SOUND TRAINING

I LIKE to say that less is more. In fact, I say it almost every day, multiple times a day, just about every time I see a client.

You see, to build defined arms, sexy legs, a flat belly, or a killer butt, you don't have to spend hours pumping iron. But you do need to do the right exercises for your goals, you need to do them correctly (or Soundly), and you need to engage your mind.

You may have heard the phrase "mind-body" before, especially if you've read books about natural healing, meditation, yoga, or relaxation. Many doctors believe that your brain is a powerful organ that can be tapped to boost immunity, strength, speed, stamina, and more.

I believe that your mind is also a powerful fitness tool, perhaps the most powerful tool you have at your disposal. Unfortunately, 95 percent of people who train don't tap into their mind power, or they tap it very little. In fact, most people disengage their minds when they work out. They watch television or other people in the gym. They daydream. They think about what they need to finish up at work, what groceries they need to buy, or what bedtime story they will read to their children at night—anything but the task at hand.

Many health clubs and trainers actually encourage this type of disengaged workout by placing televisions near treadmills, pumping out loud music, setting up reading racks and Internet connections on exercise equipment, and generally turning gyms into social meeting places. But there is a better way, one that will help you achieve the results you want faster, help you enjoy your workout more, and help you prevent discomfort and injury. That way is Sound Training.

THE IMPORTANCE OF STAYING ENGAGED

At this moment you may be thinking, "Sure, I do everything I can to distract myself from the task at hand. If I didn't, I'd never exercise."

Please don't feel guilty or inadequate. Most people do and say the same thing, usually in an attempt to entertain themselves throughout a task that they consider somewhat onerous and dull. Yet after I teach my clients how to fully engage their minds as they move their bodies, every single one of them excitedly tells me that their workouts as well as their lives have been transformed.

It is through the development of your mind-body connection that you'll learn to possess a greater sense of self. Your mind and body do speak to you, feeding you vital information about your physical, emotional, and psychological state. Honing that mind-body connection is like building

Mind Over Matter

Here are just a few examples of what some of my clients told me after they started tapping into their mind power during their workouts:

◆ "An hour goes by so quickly now, whereas before, it was all I could do to get out of the gym."

◆ "I feel better by the end of every workout. Even when I'm tired, I still go to my sessions because I know I will feel better."

◆ "I've transformed my body so quickly. I look and feel great. My workouts are so much more highly effective and targeted. The results are amazing. People tell me that I have a healthy glow."

◆ "I'm the type of person who would come up with excuses not to work out. Now it's so easy for me. My exercise sessions are a pleasure."

a perkier butt or tighter abdomen: It feels awkward in the beginning and doesn't quite make sense, but as you work at it, it all suddenly falls into place.

When you fail to hear your body's voice, you are left with uninspired workouts that bore both you and your muscles. (Yes, your muscles *do* get bored.) Boring workouts lead to inconsistency. Inconsistency leads to poor results.

Worse, failing to engage your mind before you engage your body can actually get you injured. Your body talks to you all the time. If your mind is somewhere else—whether it's the latest gossip in *People* magazine or today's guest on *Oprah*—you won't hear your body telling you: "This is enough," "This hurts," "This exercise isn't targeting the right muscle," "You've done this exercise for the past month, why not try something else?"

On the other hand, once you engage your mind, you will become at one with your workout. Think of it as Zen weight lifting. Time will flow. And you'll become fit and firm.

Here are three important reasons to engage your mind and train Soundly:

1. You'll save time. My Sound Training program will show you the most effective exercises for your individual goals as well as the most efficient methods of performing those specific exercises. You should be getting the maximum return on your fitness investment. Engaging your mind will help you maximize your results even further by helping you make every repetition count.

2. You'll stay healthy. Weight training should prevent injuries, not cause them. Many people make the mistake of waiting until something hurts before evaluating its effectiveness and safety. Unfortunately, once something hurts, it's usually too late. Tapping into your mind-body connection will help you know when a weight is too heavy or too light. It will tell you whether you're using proper form. And it will tell you when you need to modify an exercise based on your individual body mechanics. I don't believe in the "no pain, no gain" philosophy of exercise. In my method, you achieve gains through Sound Training, not pain or torture.

3. You'll feel better. When you use proper form, slow down the movement, and focus on the moment, exercise feels right. The awkwardness of exercise disappears. Instead, you feel balanced and strong. You'll look forward to your next session. You'll *feel* the difference, and you'll *see* the results. And you'll never get bored. Some people describe Zen as the ability to achieve a feeling of timelessness. You're so in the moment and so content that you don't notice time moving. Once you tap into your mind-body connection, this is how every workout will feel.

You don't *need* a trainer to train intelligently. But you do need the arsenal of information in the trainer's brain that helps him direct your workout. With my Sound Training program, you will receive the information you need to become your own trainer.

If you're a beginner, my program will help you meet your goals safely, and help you feel motivated as you do so. If you're a veteran weight lifter, my Sound Training program will give you innovative techniques and tweaks that will help jump-start a stale program, bringing you new and better results.

CONNECTING MIND AND BODY

Now that you understand why it's important to tap into your mind-body connection, I'm going to show you *how*. What follows are tips and strategies that I learned and developed after years of training hundreds of clients.

Vary your workouts. Editors from fitness magazines often interview me, and, 9 times out of 10, they want to know the 10 or so *best* moves to do in the gym. I always tell them that 10 is too small a number because it doesn't allow for variety. When every single workout is made up of the same 10 or so exercises, you start to do your workout by rote. Your mind becomes bored, your motivation plummets, and your muscles stop responding.

That's why I've offered 62 core exercises in my Sound Training program, as well as numerous tweaks on those exercises. This will allow you to make every single workout unique. Pushing yourself to do new exercises, new exercise combinations, and new variations of old exercises will keep both your mind and body engaged.

Combination workouts are at the core of my success in designing workout routines for my clients. Throughout the exercise descriptions in this chapter, I've suggested numerous combinations that have worked for me and my clients. Start with those, then add a few of your own. By changing the combinations, you can keep your workouts fresh and your motivation high. Most important, you'll experience greater results.

Don't focus on reps, focus on feel. Other exercise programs prescribe a certain number of repetitions and sets to do of each exercise. I don't. No two people are built the same. So, while 12 reps might exhaust one person's biceps, another person might need to do 20. Also, how strong you feel on Monday may change by Wednesday, so you may need to do more or fewer repetitions or sets.

Again, listen to your body. You want to work toward healthy muscle exhaustion, to your maximum perceived rate of exertion (MPRE). When you are done with a set, you should feel as if you've worked that muscle to its limit. That might happen in 10 repetitions, or 15. And it doesn't matter how long it takes you to get there, as long as you do get there.

How much weight you start with will dictate how many repetitions you can do. When deciding how much weight to lift, think about your training objectives. If you want to put on muscle size, lift more weight and do fewer repetitions. If you're after toning and sculpting, keep the repetitions higher and the pounds you lift lower.

Aim for symmetry. Many people focus on one area of their bodies and largely ignore the other areas. This results in men with huge chests and biceps and spindly chicken legs. It's time for all you guys with chicken legs to get in the gym and start doing those squats!

Sound Mind, Sound Body Success Story

I used to be a weekend runner, which meant that I would jog every Saturday and Sunday and do nothing else during the week. For many years, I knew that I needed more exercise, but I kept putting it off. I guess I was fortunate that my metabolism naturally allowed me to maintain my weight for the past 20 years despite horrible eating and exercise habits.

My wife gave me a gift certificate to a sports club one year as a gift. For me, that broke the ice to working out. I liked the trainer I worked with at this club, but I hated the crowds. It seemed as if 15 to 20 people were always there who knew me from my restaurants. I could never get any peace.

So I switched to the smaller, quieter atmosphere of the Madison Square Club and began training with David. He showed me an entirely new way to think about training, making me much more aware of my body. It was a very new thing for me to spend 3 or more days a week in front of a mirror for an hour at a time. David helped me to see that using proper form in an exercise or stretch means first picturing it in my mind and then focusing on the muscle I want to use as I perform the exercise.

Before I started training with David, I had suffered a rotator cuff injury and had to give up tennis because of it. David showed me how to strengthen the muscles around my shoulder. Now I can play tennis for hours without pain.

—Danny Meyer

There is nothing more beautiful than a symmetrical body, where all of the muscles are equally firm. Michelangelo's David is a visual masterpiece—symmetrical from head to toe. When designing routines for my clients, I try to keep in mind their specific body genetics as well as their overall goals. Regardless of their requests, I never lose sight of the need to create one flowing line of physical symmetry. All of the pieces of the

When Your Body Hurts

If you've ever watched children on a playground, you can easily find yourself mourning your body of yesteryear. Children can do all sorts of crazy stunts, from jumping off seesaws to rolling on hard dirt to tripping and falling on their faces. Yet despite the tears and screams, they usually get up and within minutes are running around pain-free.

I don't know about you, but if I tried to run around like that today, I'd hear a series of complaints from my body. What happened?

For me, years of improper weight lifting during my adolescence did a number on my neck. For you, it might not even be exercise-related. Maybe you were in a car accident. Or you might have sprained your ankle while getting off a bus. Or maybe parts of your body just hurt and you don't know why. Whatever the reasons, you must address those concerns when lifting weights. Otherwise, those nagging aches and pains will destroy your workouts. Your workouts could even make your aches and pains worse.

I've listed the most common parts of the body where people experience discomfort, along with tips and exercise modifications to address your concerns.

Knees

If you've ever injured your knee, you should take special precautions, even if your knee is currently pain-free. For all standing movements, pay extra-careful attention to sitting back into your heels so that the force of the movement drives through the backs of your legs and not forward into your knees.

Before doing leg exercises, warm up your knee area first by doing your first few movements without weight, just going through the motion. If you experience any discomfort, limit your range of motion, for example, by doing partial leg extensions.

If you can do a squat, do so with a wide stance and don't lock your knees. If you still feel knee pain, avoid squats and instead focus on leg extensions (making sure not to lock out at the top of the movement), leg curls, and floor work.

puzzle must fit together, or else it doesn't work.

That's one reason I recommend a total-body workout. Here's another. Many people are stronger on one side of their body than the other.

Throughout the exercises, I offer tips on isolating one side of your body at a time, helping you close the gap between that initial imbalance. It is also one reason I prefer dumbbells over barbells and machines: They

Lower Back

Strengthening your lower abdominals with Reverse Crunches will go a long way toward reducing your back pain (so will stretching your hamstrings). But you need to be careful when doing crunches. Limit your range of motion, especially if you experience any lower-back discomfort, and consider squeezing a large exercise ball between your calves and thighs to prevent your back from arching during the move.

Before doing any back exercises, make sure to warm up by stretching your back as though you were a cat. During all exercises, pay careful attention to keeping your abs tight. And avoid any overhead movements and squats, which are difficult to perform without arching your back.

Shoulder

Before each session, warm up your shoulders and rotator cuff area with the appropriate stretches. I like to do windmills with my arms out to the sides performing small circular rotations both forward and backward. You can also do these with your arms extended in front of you, parallel to the floor. Bend over and allow one arm to hang down at a time. Pretend there's a weight in your hand, pulling your arm downward. Slowly rotate your hand clockwise and then counterclockwise. Then swing it forward and back in a pendulum movement. Follow up with a series of dumbbell rows either with no weight or with very light resistance.

Avoid overhead presses, and instead opt for Side Laterals and Front Raises. Avoid bench presses and flies, and instead do modified pushups (not all the way), making sure your chest is over your hands on the descent.

Neck

Developing your trapezius muscles will help support your neck, so shoulder shrugs should be a part of your program. You also want to strengthen your rhomboids with prone rows to improve your posture, taking the tension out of your neck. Instead of doing the rows while standing, do them while lying prone on a bench, and raise the dumbbells only as high as is comfortable.

allow you to isolate each side of your body.

Protect your joints. When doing any exercise, your knees and elbows should always be loose, about 95 percent extended at the most. But that doesn't mean they should flop around. Even though your knees and elbows will always be slightly bent, they should be firm and fixed in place. The one exception to this is your wrists. Lock them.

Don't show off. Many people sacrifice form in their zeal to lift

The Right Moves for You

Refer to this chart when designing your program to help you pick the best exercises for your body type. As you will see, a few moves appear in more than one category. That largely depends on how you do them. If you do the move with low reps and high weight, it's a strength move. If you do it with low weight and high reps, it's a sculpting move.

CHEST
STRENGTH MOVES
- Standard Pushup (p. 45)
- Incline Pushup (p. 46)
- Standard Dumbbell Bench Press (p. 47)
- Incline Dumbbell Bench Press (p. 48)
- Decline Dumbbell Bench Press (p. 49)

SHAPING/TONING MOVES
- Dumbbell Fly (p. 50)
- Incline Dumbbell Fly (p. 52)
- Decline Dumbbell Fly (p. 52)

LEGS
STRENGTH MOVES
- Squat/Knee Bend (p. 54)
- Plié Squat (no Calf Raise) (p. 55)
- Wall Squat with Ball (p. 56)
- Stiff-Leg Dead Lift (p. 57)
- Partial Dead Lift (p. 58)
- Standing Calf Raise (p. 59)
- Leg Extension (p. 60)
- Leg Curl (p. 61)
- Prone Leg Curl (p. 62)
- David's Deluxe Floor Routine (p. 64)

SHAPING/TONING MOVES
- Plié Squat with Calf Raise (p. 55)
- Stiff-Leg Dead Lift (p. 57)
- David's Reverse Prone Scissors (p. 63)
- David's Deluxe Lunge Routine (p. 66)
- David's Donkey Deluxe (p. 68)
- Frog Jump (p. 70)
- David's Crab Crawl (p. 71)
- David's Platypus Walk (p. 72)
- Pelvic Tilt (p. 73)
- Bench Stepup with Kick and Extension (p. 74)

BACK
STRENGTH MOVES
- One-Arm Dumbbell Row (p. 76)
- Bent-Over Dumbbell Row (p. 77)
- Under-Handed Dumbbell Row (p. 78)

heavier weights. Once a weight becomes too heavy for you to lift, you end up jerking your body, losing the fluidity that is so important. You also tend to lose proper body alignment. Think form first, heft second.

Look, feel, and touch. I like my clients to do their exercises in front of a mirror. That way they can *look* at their form to make sure their shoulders are retracted, their back is flat, and their joints are loose. Then, I ask them to visualize the move-

- ◆ Pullover (p. 79)
- ◆ Superman (p. 80)
- ◆ Good Morning (p. 81)

SHAPING/TONING MOVES
- ◆ One-Arm Dumbbell Row (p. 76)
- ◆ Good Morning (p. 81)

SHOULDERS

STRENGTH MOVES
- ◆ Military/Shoulder Press (p. 83)
- ◆ Side Lateral (p. 84)
- ◆ Front Raise (p. 85)
- ◆ David's Press (p. 86)
- ◆ Shrug (p. 87)

SHAPING/TONING MOVES
- ◆ Side Lateral (p. 84)
- ◆ Front Raise (p. 85)
- ◆ David's "The Chicken" (p. 88)

ARMS

STRENGTH MOVES
- ◆ Biceps Curl (p. 90)
- ◆ Forearm Raise (p. 91)
- ◆ Incline Biceps Curl (p. 92)
- ◆ Hammer Curl (p. 93)
- ◆ Reverse-Grip Curl (p. 93)

- ◆ Skull Crusher (p. 94)
- ◆ Upright Triceps Overhead Extension (p. 96)
- ◆ Dips on a Bench (p. 97)

SHAPING/TONING MOVES
- ◆ Concentration Curl (p. 92)
- ◆ Triceps Kickback (p. 95)
- ◆ David's Reverse Crab (p. 98)
- ◆ Reverse-Grip Pushup (p. 99)

ABS

SHAPING/TONING MOVES
- ◆ Basic Crunch (p. 101)
- ◆ Oblique Crunch (p. 102)
- ◆ Reverse Crunch (p. 103)
- ◆ African Dance Step (p. 104)
- ◆ Oblique Twist (p. 104)
- ◆ Torso Turn (p. 105)
- ◆ Scissors Reverse Crunch (p. 106)
- ◆ Leg Circles (p. 107)
- ◆ David's Isometric Ab (p. 108)
- ◆ Bicycle (p. 110)

CARDIO-SCULPTING MOVES
- ◆ Shadowboxing (p. 112)
- ◆ Kicks (p. 114)

ment and *feel* of the exercise. Finally, they actually perform the move, all the while looking at their form and feeling the movement, engaging the right muscles. I even have them physically *touch* the muscle they intend to target with their fingers to make sure it feels taut. If you do the same, you'll be able to subconsciously police your body mechanics throughout every move, making small adjustments that will increase the effectiveness.

Make the top and bottom count. Many people rest when they get to the top or bottom of an exercise, such as the up position of a bench press or the down position of a dumbbell row. I ask my clients to instead make the most of the movement here by squeezing the muscle they are working. This isometric contraction will give you an extra burn, maximizing your results. Squeeze, don't snooze, at the top of the movement.

Stay in touch with your goals. The same exercises that help your friend stay and look fit may not do the same for you simply because you may have different goals and issues. If your friend is an apple, she will need to focus on her abs and her back. If you're a pear, however, you'll need to pay attention to your inner and outer thighs and your glutes. In the program section of this chapter, I'll explain how to design your program for your specific needs. No two people are the same; no two people want the same results; no two people should complete exactly the same workout.

THE SIX ESSENTIALS OF EXERCISE

Tapping into your mind-body connection is a key component of my program, but it's not the only unique aspect. In all, my program is based on six key concepts. As I describe each exercise and explain how to construct your program, I'll come back to these key concepts over and over again.

1. Body mechanics. Proper posture is the foundation of every strength-training move. In fact, good posture should be the foundation of every move you make at work, at home, and on your weight bench.

The basic posture for every single exercise in my program is the same. To learn it, stand up and focus your attention on your belly. Contract your abs and suck them in. At the same time, contract your glutes. When you do this, your pelvis should tip back, flattening and supporting your lower back. Pay attention to your hips. Are you tilting them too far forward, causing a swayed back? If so, bring them back into alignment with your body. (Many models come to me with this problem—the result of years on the runway.)

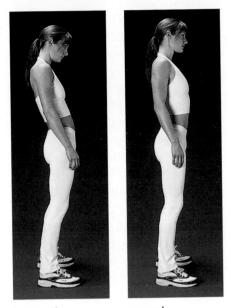

incorrect   correct

Now, focus on your feet. Bring your weight back into your heels and away from the balls. Focus on your shoulder blades. Retract them and pull them close together, expanding your chest. Focus on your head. Is it aligned with your body, or scrunched up or tilting to one side? Bring it into alignment.

There. That's good posture. Now close your eyes and mentally feel your posture. Feel your balance, your relaxation, your centeredness, your breathing. If you've practiced yoga, this is the fundamental "mountain pose." And it's the foundation for every single exercise in my program.

2. Concentration. When you train intelligently, you slow everything down and stay in the moment. You concentrate on the motion and feel of the exercise. Focus on the muscle you are working: Can you feel the movement and warmth there? Focus on your body mechanics: Are you balanced, strong, and centered? Focus on the muscles you are *not* working: Are they relaxed? Feel the movement of the exercise. Go slowly. Stay in the moment. Breathe. If you lose your focus, stop, then start again. When performed correctly, my workouts are physically, spiritually, and emotionally balancing and uplifting.

3. Flow. Done correctly, strength training should feel like meditation or yoga. You should feel as if you are moving fluidly with your breath. That means you must slow the movement down, breathing in as you lengthen your muscles (usually when lowering a weight) and breathing out when you contract your muscles (usually when raising a weight.) The slower you go, the more resistance you apply through the movement, making your burn more efficient.

4. Visualization. Your mind is closely connected to every movement your body makes. I'll often tell you to put your brain in your butt or belly button or shoulder blade or whatever part of your body on which I want you to concentrate. If you are visualizing the move and the area you are moving, every repetition works. You squeeze, engage, and contract the right muscles, not the wrong ones. For example, let's say you're doing an exercise for your legs. If you feel your face burning, the veins in your neck are about to explode, and your arms feel as if you just did a series of biceps curls, you weren't focusing on isolating the movement in the body part that you want to work.

5. Gaze. Where you look and what you look at during a move can make all the difference in doing the move right or doing it wrong. For example, when you look down while doing a squat, you'll round your shoulders and risk hurting your back. But if you keep your gaze straight ahead, you'll more easily remain in the proper body position.

6. Attitude. Too often, people skip exercises or fail to do them correctly because of two little evil words: "I can't." You are able or not able to do what you believe you can or can't do. Choose to believe in yourself. Trust your body. It's capable of more than you think.

WHAT YOU'LL NEED

To get stronger, you have numerous tools at your disposal, from rubber tubes to machines to body weight to dumbbells. For most of the exercises in my program, you'll be using dumbbells.

Compared to other types of resistance, dumbbells most support your mind-body connection. They allow you the mobility and flexibility you need to tweak an exercise to your body's specific needs. It's so much easier to adjust your body position with a pair of dumbbells as opposed to a more cumbersome bar or exercise machine.

Also, we all have a dominant side. Dumbbells allow you to address strength imbalances by forcing you to lift with one side of your body at a time. They are also the most convenient and affordable type of equipment you can buy for home exercise.

I recommend that you start with a series of dumbbells ranging from 2 to 25 pounds. And men, don't automatically opt for the heaviest weights you think you can lift. For some of the moves I suggest—such as lateral raises—even the strongest guys need to use fairly light weights. In addition to dumbbells, you'll also need a good adjustable weight bench that you can set at both an incline and a decline. Adjustable weight benches can be expensive. If you're on a budget, you can get by with a less expensive flat bench by propping one end up on a sturdy box or aerobics step.

You'll also need ankle weights, and I strongly recommend you purchase either a pullup bar or a squat rack. You will find a large exercise ball and small medicine ball useful, too. (For tips on buying equipment, see "Outfitting Your Home Gym" on page 11.)

Though dumbbells form the core of my program, you will also be doing exercises such as pushups, abdominal crunches, and dips that use your body weight for resistance. These core moves are the fundamental exercises we learned in grade school; they help create a strong platform from which your advanced moves will be performed.

THE SOUND TRAINING PROGRAM

I've organized the exercises in my program into three main areas: strength moves, shaping/toning moves, and cardio sculpting.

Strength moves. These exercises will help you build muscle, your body's calorie-burning furnace. Each pound of muscle burns between 35 and 50 calories a day just to maintain itself. The more muscle you have, the faster your metabolism. I've grouped them according to the major muscle groups, including your back, chest, butt, shoulders, arms, legs, and abs. Some of these exercises have been around for a long time, and you'll find many of them in other weight-lifting books. What you won't find in those books is what I bring to them: the mind-body connection. I've described how to fully engage your mind, helping you to better direct the movement of your body. I've also alerted you to what you shouldn't feel during an exercise, and how to correct the problem.

Shaping/toning moves. These exercises do just that—shape and tone your muscles. Shaping and toning make the difference between forming the bulky muscles of a football player and the sinewy, shapely muscles of a dancer. The philosophy is simple: To shape and tone, one must lower the weight, increase the number of repetitions, and do those specific moves that focus on the smaller muscle fibers of each muscle group. For example, Dumbbell Flies for the chest, One-Arm Dumbbell Rows for the back, and Plié Squats with Calf Raises for the legs and glutes.

Cardio sculpting. I include this series of exercises for clients who want long, firm muscles, but don't want to call attention to themselves. In other words, they don't want to look as if they live at the gym; they want to look as if the gym rounds out their lives. For example, supermodel Heidi Klum, the star of my "Bikini Boot Camp" on page 228, does only cardio sculpting. These moves help you shape your body as well as burn hundreds of extra calories during your workout, so you can do them as a great aerobic burn for a few minutes between your core moves, or you can completely focus your workout on cardio sculpting. It just depends on your personal goals.

(continued on page 42)

David's Stretches

Five to 10 minutes of stretching before and after you lift weights will keep your muscles supple and prevent injury. It will also help you to feel good. A flexible body is an energetic body.

As with weight lifting, you want to stretch your entire body. You'll enjoy stretching more if you flow through your stretching moves, advancing fluidly from one stretch into the next. Start with your standing stretches, then do your sitting stretches, and then your prone stretches. Always stretch after a warmup, when your body is warm. Here are some of my favorites.

Calf stretch. Stand with one foot 2 to 3 feet in front of the other. Rest your hands on top of a sturdy table. Bend your front leg as you extend your rear leg and angle your body forward so that it forms a straight line from your rear ankle to your extended arms.

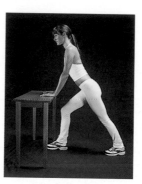

Chest stretch. Clasp both hands behind your back, retract your shoulder blades, and open your chest. Raise your hands as high as you can behind your back without allowing your shoulders to scrunch upward toward your ears or to slouch forward. Lower your hands and then interlace your fingers and repeat.

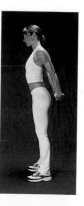

Upper-back stretch. Bring your hands forward, pushing your palms forward in front of your chest as you round your upper back and lower your chin toward your chest.

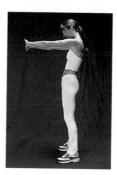

Shoulder stretch. Bring up your left arm so your bicep is near your ear. Bend your arm so that your forearm and hand are behind your right shoulder. With your right hand, pull your elbow slightly closer to your head to increase the stretch. Make sure to keep your head aligned, not cocked to one side.

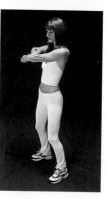

Groin stretch. Sit on the floor with the bottoms of your feet pressed together. Allow your knees to drop to the sides. Hold on to the tops of your feet, using your hands to pull your pelvis forward, flattening your back. To increase the stretch, bend forward slightly, keeping your back flat.

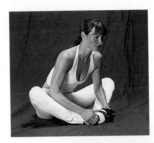

Hamstring stretch. Extend one leg, keeping the other bent from the groin stretch. Slowly lean forward from your waist, making sure to keep your back flat as you lower your abdomen to your thigh. Repeat on the other side.

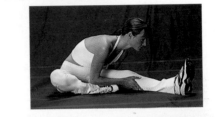

Thigh stretch. Lie on one side with your bottom leg extended. Prop your head on your hand for comfort. Bend your top leg, bringing your top foot toward your buttocks, grasping it with your top hand.

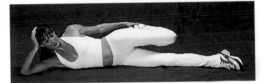

Lower-back stretch. Roll onto your back and hug your knees into your chest, allowing your body to rock gently.

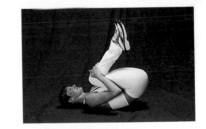

Buttocks stretch. Extend your left leg and bend your right leg so your right calf is parallel to the floor. While keeping your back and shoulders flat on the floor, cross your left leg over your right leg. Keep your left shoulder on the floor. Repeat on the other side.

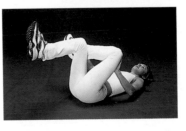

In addition to those standard exercises, I've also provided a number of other exclusive exercises that I've tweaked and developed over the years in response to the needs of my clients. Each of my clients has specific needs and physiological concerns, so I have found specific ways to tweak each exercise to make it distinctively theirs. If it's a completely new move that I discovered and developed, I've labeled it "David's Signature Move." Because many of these moves use your body weight for resistance, these moves are perfect when you're traveling and don't have your dumbbells. Other special features of my program include Distinctively David tips, which will help you boost the effectiveness of the moves, prevent injury, and generally increase your enjoyment and motivation; advanced moves that require a good strength foundation, balance, agility, or all three (if you are a beginner, don't try these moves until week 3 or later. Wait until you feel comfortable with the standard moves before moving onto advanced moves); "Try This" exercises that list my favorite exercise combinations; and body type icons that you should refer to when designing your program to make sure an exercise is right for you—many of the moves are great for all body types, but some are not. (See "Your Program" on page 116 for specifics on how to adapt my program for *you*.)

For all of the exercises in the sections that follow, which are organized by the body part or region you want to work, I not only give you the nuts and bolts of how to perform the exercise but also tell you where to feel the movement. (If the name of the muscle is unfamiliar to you, check out "Muscle Gallery.") That's important. When you can feel the exercise, you do it better. What happens if you don't feel the movement in the same area that I ask you to focus? That means you are either using bad form or not fully taking advantage of your mind-body connection.

SOUND TRAINING TIPS

◆ Always warm up. Never lift when your muscles are cold. Before your exercise session, warm up by running, walking, or doing some other form of cardiovascular exercise for 5 to 10 minutes. If it's cold outside or if you are feeling tired, warm up for 10 to 15 minutes. Listen to your body. When your muscles feel warm and pliable, you're ready to lift weights. In addition to getting your heart rate up, you also want to pump blood into the area that you will be working first. If you are starting with your chest, back, or shoulders, do a series of shoulder rotations and then some side laterals and front raises with very light weight. For your back, also add some Cat Stretches. If you are starting with your legs, do a series of partial squats without weight. And for your first few exercises, start with a weight that is slightly lighter than you could probably lift, and advance to a set of heavier resistance.

◆ Perform all of the dumbbell moves slowly and methodically, making your ascent and descent last 3 to 5 seconds each. On the descent, hold the dumbbells 2 to 3 inches above your body, maintaining a maximum contraction in the muscle group you are working.

◆ Add in some cardio. For best results, you should combine your weight-lifting program with 30 to 45 minutes of cardiovascular exercise such as power walking or rowing twice a week or more, especially if you are trying to lose weight. In the programs section of this chapter, you'll find suggested cardio moves for your body type.

◆ Stretch. A side effect of building a stronger body is that your muscles will contract and tighten. So you want to stretch after every session to lengthen them. See "David's Stretches" on page 40.

Muscle Gallery

If you're like most people, you know where your abdominal muscles are located, but you might not be as familiar with other muscles and muscle groups. Here's a quick rundown of the muscles you'll be working in the Sound Training program.

Abdominals (abs): Stomach
Abductors: Outer thighs
Adductors: Inner thighs
Biceps: Front of upper arms
Deltoids: Shoulders
Erector spinae: Lower back and spine
Gastrocnemius: Calves
Glutes: Buttocks
Hamstrings: Back of thighs
Latissimus dorsi (lats): Mid- and lower back

Levator scapulae (shoulder blades): Engage the lats
Obliques: Sides of the abdomen
Pectoralis major (pectorals, or pecs): Chest
Quadriceps (quads): Front of thighs
Rectus abdominis: Front of the abdomen
Rhomboids: Upper back
Soleus: Lower calves
Transverse abdominis: Pulls in the belly
Trapezius (traps): Neck and shoulders
Triceps: Back of upper arms

CHEST

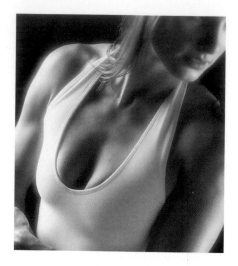

Your chest is made up of a pair of large muscles called your pectoralis major, or pecs. Running along your collar bone, breast bone, and ribs, your pecs help you push and press. When doing any of the chest movements, whether it's a bench press or a pushup, your body position and focus is the same. Follow these general pointers.

Stabilize your core. Your core is your foundation. If you built a house on a weak foundation, it would wash away in the first storm. Your body is the same. Your butt, back, and abs form your core. Contracting your abs and butt and supporting your back will keep your body in position for each exercise.

Retract your shoulder blades. If you roll your shoulders forward in any chest exercise, you risk placing undue stress on your shoulders. Before doing any lifting, first make sure that your shoulder blades are retracted and pulled close together. This will open your chest, the primary muscle being engaged in the exercises.

Lock your wrists. You want your wrists locked in position and aligned with your elbows, not rolled backward or forward.

Perform slow, smooth movements. This is true for all exercises, but especially so with chest motions. I don't know how many guys I've seen bouncing barbells off their chests in order to get enough momentum to push it up. This not only reduces the effectiveness of the exercise, it's also dangerous. In my Sound Training program, you will perform each rep in a smooth and controlled manner. This will maximize the burn and the effectiveness of the exercise.

◇ ◇ ◉ ◇ ✦

standard pushup | pectoralis major, triceps

a. With your hands directly under your chest, inhale as you lower your chest toward your hands, making sure to keep your abs tight and your back flat.

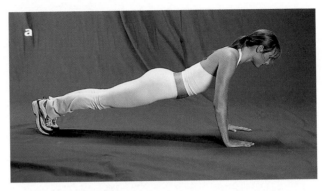

b. Once you reach the floor, press up as you exhale. Concentrate on pressing through your chest muscles. When you reach the top of the pushup, extend your arms but keep your elbows loose. This is where my method of visualization is essential. You need to put your brain in your chest throughout this movement. You do not want to feel the movement in your shoulders or lower back. If you feel this in your shoulders, your hand placement is wrong. Check to make sure your hands are directly under your chest.

If your lower back is bothering you, you are probably slouching. Check your alignment, lock your hips, and tighten your abs. Last, if your elbows hurt, you are locking them out; remember to keep them loose throughout the movement. If you don't have enough strength to push yourself up, start by doing pushups on your knees or against a bar or something stationary.

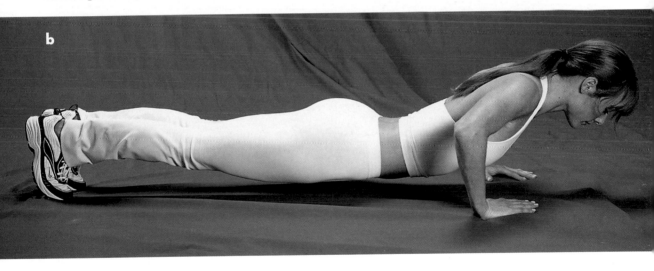

◆ **Distinctively David**

During the pushup, retract your shoulder blades, pulling them down your back. This simple move will immediately open and engage your chest, preventing you from overworking the trapezius and deltoid muscles (see "Muscle Gallery" on page 43) in your neck and shoulders.

incline pushup | pectoralis major

With your hands on the floor, prop the balls of your feet up on your bench and stabilize your torso so that your back is flat and your abs are tight. With this move, it's especially important to keep your abs tight because gravity will attempt to pull your hips down. Inhale as you lower your chest toward the floor, making sure to keep your abs tight and back flat throughout the move. Exhale as you press back up, squeezing your chest muscles.

　　If your lower back is bothering you, you are probably slouching. Check your alignment, lock your hips, and tighten your abs.

◆Try This

For the ultimate pushup experience, try my Deluxe Pushup Routine. Place yourself in an incline pushup position with your hands slightly wider than shoulder-width apart and perform a set to exhaustion. Take a 10-second rest and then move your hands closer together. Perform another set to exhaustion. For the final set, place your hands close together, but at an angle with your fingers pointing toward each other. (These are called Close-Grip Pushups.) You can also try doing standard pushups with one hand elevated on a step or dumbbell 3 to 6 inches higher than the other hand (called Asymmetrical Pushups). Last, for the ultimate burn, place both hands on a medicine ball, steady your core by keeping your abs tight, and perform the pushups. The most advanced pushup move of the lot, this medicine ball exercise requires strength, agility, and coordination.

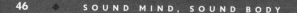

◇ ◇ ◆ ◇ ◇ ✦

standard dumbbell bench press | pectoralis major, triceps

a. Lie on your back on a bench and hold a pair of dumbbells end to end near chest level. Press your lower back into the bench and pinch your shoulder blades together. For greater lower-back protection and core stability, rest your feet on the bench.

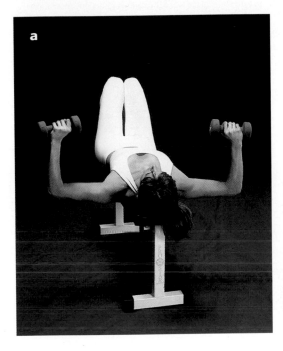

b. Exhale as you press the dumbbells up and slightly forward. Fully extend your arms, but don't lock your elbows. Inhale as you lower the dumbbells to your chest.

Note: You can isolate your triceps with this move by using a slightly narrower grip and employing your mind-body connection to press up through your triceps rather than your chest. If that aggravates shoulder pain, however, lower the dumbbells only partway. If your mind-body connection is awake, you'll know when you can't go any farther.

If you feel this move in your shoulders, you may be rolling your shoulders forward, locking your elbows, not retracting your shoulder blades, not pressing the dumbbell directly above your chest, not locking your wrists, or lowering the dumbbell too far.

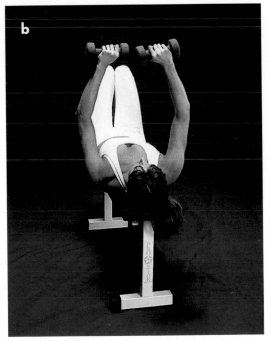

◆ Distinctively David

Make sure your torso is stable by contracting your abs and pressing your lower back into the bench, and retracting your shoulder blades. This will allow you to maximize the benefit to your chest and take away potential shoulder strain.

incline dumbbell bench press | upper pectoralis major

a. Adjust your bench so that the seat is at a 45- to 60-degree angle. Sit down and hold a pair of dumbbells end to end just above your chest. Firmly press your buttocks and back against the back of the bench.

b. Keep your abs firm and exhale as you raise both dumbbells up and slightly forward, concentrating on squeezing your chest muscles. Extend your arms, but don't lock your elbows. Inhale as you slowly lower the dumbbells to your chest. To increase the difficulty, try raising just one dumbbell at a time.

   Note: Incline presses are not for everyone. If you have shoulder problems, limit your range of motion. Remember: Persistent pain leads to injury, not gain.

◆**Distinctively David**
To make sure you press up correctly, look straight ahead as you lift the weights and bring the weights into your field of vision.

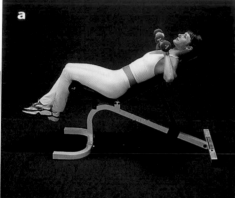

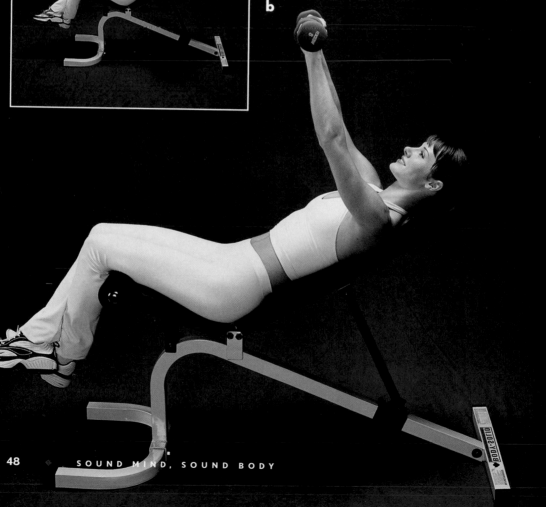

decline dumbbell bench press | lower pectoralis major

a. Adjust your bench into a decline position, with the angle set at 45 to 60 degrees. Lie on the bench so that your head is closer to the floor. Hold a pair of dumbbells end to end just above your chest.

b. Exhale and press the dumbbells up and slightly forward toward your lower chest. Throughout the move, keep your abs tight and your back flat. As you press up, squeeze your lower chest muscles.

   Pay particular attention to your back during this move. Make sure your abs are tight, keeping your back from arching. If you need additional lower-back support, place one leg on top of the bench, giving your lower back greater stability.

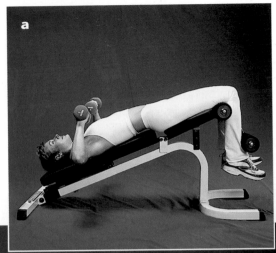

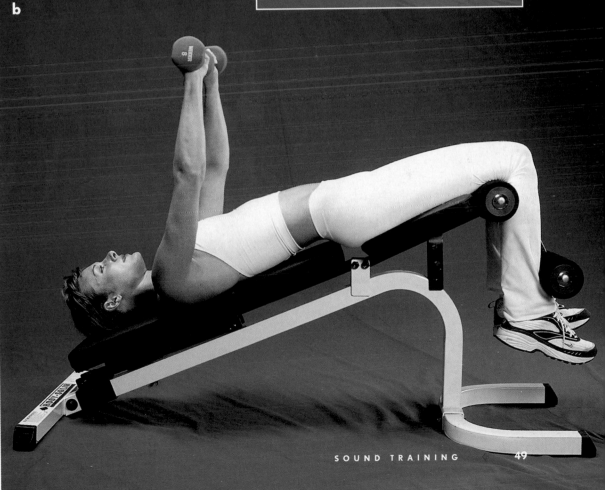

◇ ◆ ◗ ◆ ✪

dumbbell fly | pectoralis major

Flies are great toning and shaping exercises that will address the outer part of the chest area.

a. Lie on your back on your bench. Hold the dumbbells above your chest with your palms facing each other. Press your shoulders and back down against the bench.

b. With your abs and back firm, inhale as you bring the dumbbells out to the sides, leading with your elbows. Your arms should be slightly bent to keep the stress off your joints. Stop when the dumbbells reach the plane of your body. Exhale as you squeeze through your chest and press from your elbows to bring the dumbbells back up.

　Note: When pressing the dumbbells on top, make sure they are over the middle top of your chest. (The old school had you holding the dumbbells above your collarbone, which posed a greater risk of injury to your rotator cuff area.) If you have any shoulder problems, do not do these presses.

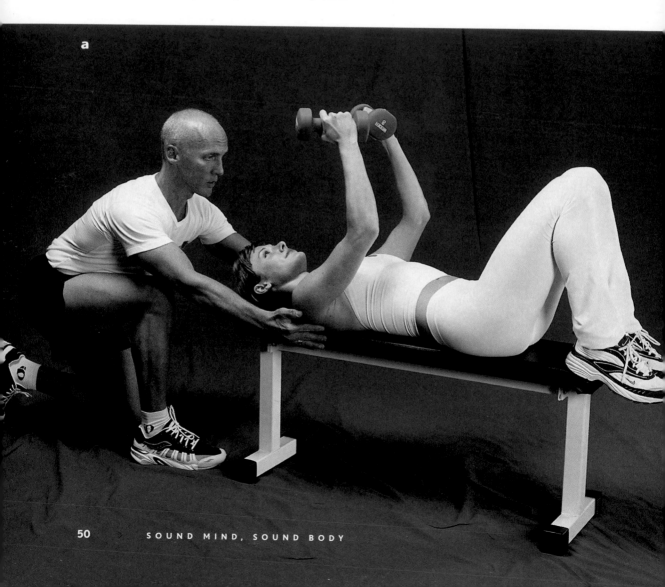

a

◆ Distinctively David

Even though your arms are bent throughout this exercise, they are still locked in position. Keep your arms firm throughout the move, and focus on squeezing your chest muscles. Also, as I'm squeezing up, I like to slightly turn my hands forward, bringing my pinkies in and the front heads of the dumbbells together. That will give you a greater lower-chest contraction. Looking slightly forward will help guide the dumbbells into their proper position.

◆ Try This—Advanced

I like to do a combination move that I call the Advanced Incline Dumbbell Fly Press. It truly is advanced. Make sure you are comfortable with both moves before combining them. You can do the dumbbell fly first, which will "pre-exhaust" your chest for the press (see "The Right Combination" on page 115 for other combination moves). Or you can do the press first, moving into the fly.

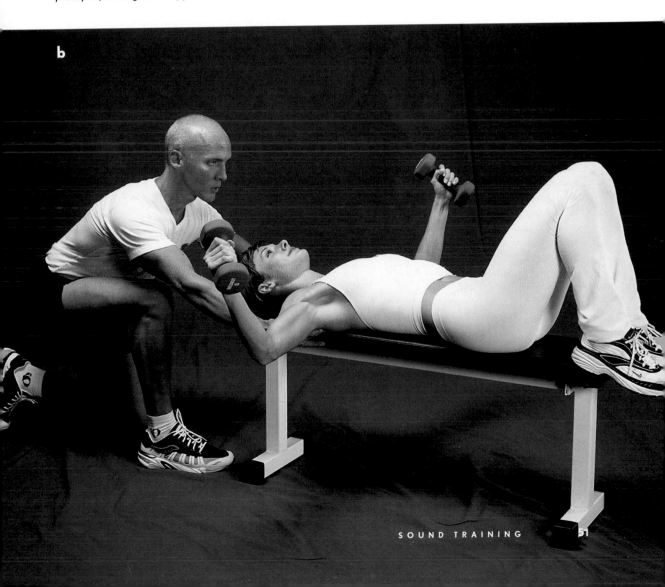

b

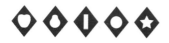

incline dumbbell fly | upper pectoralis major | ADVANCED

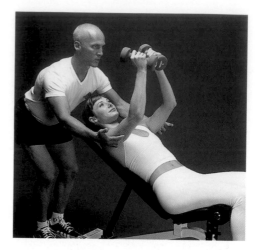

Adjust your bench so that the seat is at a 45- to 60-degree angle. Sit down and hold a pair of dumbbells above your chest with your palms facing each other. Firmly press your buttocks and back against the back of the bench. Keep your abs firm. Inhale as you bring the dumbbells out to the sides, leading with your elbows. Your arms should be slightly bent to keep the stress off your joints. Stop when the dumbbells reach the plane of your body. Then exhale as you squeeze through your chest and press from your elbows to bring the dumbbells back up.

Note: If you have shoulder problems, limit your range of motion or skip this exercise altogether.

decline dumbbell fly | lower pectoralis major | ADVANCED

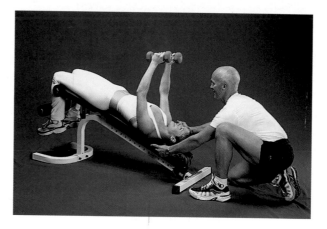

Adjust your bench into a decline position, with the angle set at 45 to 60 degrees. Lie on the bench so that your head is closer to the floor. Hold a pair of dumbbells with your arms extended above your chest. Inhale as you lower the dumbbells out to the sides, making sure to keep them in the same plane as your chest and not allowing gravity to pull them toward your collarbone. Exhale as you press them back toward your lower chest. Throughout the move, keep your abs tight and your back flat.

◆Try This—Advanced

This superset move is meant for you men and women who really want to pump up your chest routine. It's extremely advanced. First, perform a set of Decline Dumbbell Flies followed immediately by a set of Decline Dumbbell Bench Presses (see page 49). (Use more weight for the presses than you do for the flies.) Then, with the same weight that you used for the presses, do a set of Pullovers (see page 79) with your bench set in a decline position. You can interchange the flies and presses, but I generally like to do the presses first. The pullovers can also follow the presses, in which case the flies would follow the pullovers.

LEGS

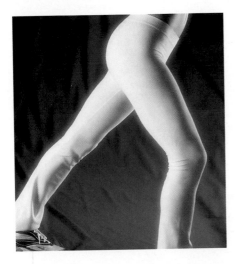

Your legs are the largest and strongest muscle group in your body. They need to be strong to support the rest of your body as you walk. That's why the average strong man can lift 2 times his body weight with his legs, compared to only 1 to 1½ times with his upper body.

For shapely legs, you need to work some key areas: your glutes (buttocks), your hamstrings (the muscles that form the rear of your thighs), and your quadriceps (the muscles that form the front of your thighs). Depending on your goals, you might also pay attention to your adductors (your inner thighs) and your abductors (your outer thighs) as well as your calves.

Again, stabilize! Because many leg movements, such as squats and lunges, require standing while holding weight, you must keep your core stable throughout the movements by keeping your abs and glutes tight. If you don't have a stable core, you can lose your balance or stress your lower back.

Use your heels. When doing any standing leg exercise, focus on your feet, keeping your weight in your heels. Your heels are your anchors, and they're the source of your drive. If you drive up through your heels, your power will transfer into your hamstrings and then into your glutes. On the other hand, if you stand with your weight in the balls of your feet, you'll not only feel unstable, but also you'll transfer the power into your knees. That's dangerous. And it's not an efficient use of your power.

Isolate the muscles. As your legs generally make up your strongest muscle group, pay careful attention to isolating the specific leg area that you are trying to engage. Without focusing on isolating the movement, it will be too easy to cheat your way through the move and not get the most benefit from the exercise.

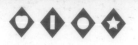

squat/knee bend | quadriceps, glutes, hamstrings

a. Stand with your feet shoulder-width apart. Make sure your weight is equally balanced on both feet, your core is stable, your shoulder blades are retracted, and your eyes are focused straight ahead. Clasp a dumbbell with both hands between your legs. (If you're a beginner, do this move—called a knee bend—without weight first.)

b. Bring your body weight back to your heels, and as you inhale, squat down while pushing your butt out, allowing your back to arch slightly. Stop when your thighs are parallel to the floor. Exhale as you push through your heels and squeeze your buttocks to rise up.

If you have had knee surgery or knee injuries, squats are probably not the best option for you. If you experience pain in your knees, you're probably putting your body weight on the balls of your feet instead of your heels. If your lower back hurts, either you are arching your back too much or your abs are not tight enough.

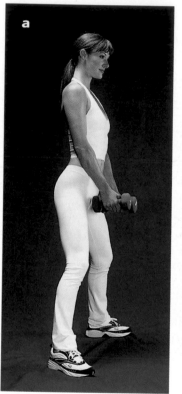

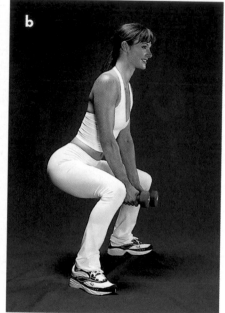

◆Distinctively David

Squats are not always the best choice for women since they can lead to thicker butts and hips. To prevent that, make this simple adjustment. Widen your stance and turn your toes out to a plié position at a 45-degree angle, so that your feet are slightly wider than shoulder-width apart. That simple tweak will put the focus more on your inner thighs and your glutes. Knee strength permitting, you can also take a close stance with your feet 3 to 4 inches apart. This will blast your quads.

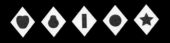

plié squat with calf raise | glutes, adductors, gastrocnemius, soleus | ADVANCED

Get in a squat position with your feet shoulder-width apart and hold a dumbbell between your legs. Your toes should be turned out at a 45-degree angle. Stick your butt back as you squat down, keeping your body weight in your heels. As you are sinking into the squat, bring your heels off the ground and rise onto the balls of your feet. (Continue to keep your body weight back toward your heels.) Then, bring your heels back to the floor and shift your body weight back into them, squeezing your inner thighs and glutes before pressing back up.

Pay attention to your knees and lower back with this move. Don't allow your knees to jut beyond your toes. Also, don't lock them in the "up" position. If you lower back hurts, you are not keeping your abs tight enough throughout the move.

This can also be performed with someone (as shown), allowing greater stability and more range of motion.

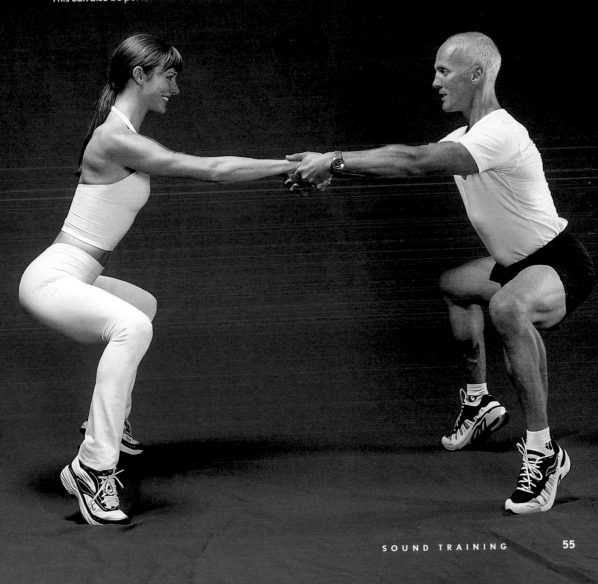

wall squat with ball | glutes, quadriceps, hamstrings

Place an exercise ball between your back and a wall, leaning into it so that the ball rests at the base of your spine. Bring your feet about 12 inches in front of you and keep them shoulder-width apart. Squat down slowly until your thighs are parallel to the floor. Hold for 2 to 3 seconds and then press through your heels to rise. Throughout the move, keep your knees loose. On your last rep, hold the squat position with your thighs parallel to the floor for 20 seconds to 1 minute.

If your knees hurt, check to make sure that they are not jutting beyond your toes.

◆ Try This—Advanced

You can turn any squat or lunge into a plyometric move (an exercise to increase muscle power) by adding a leap. Plyometrics are great if you play sports that require running, cutting movements, or jumping, but they are advanced. Don't do them if you have knee or back problems. Here are two:

1. *Leaping squats. Get in a squat position and hold a dumbbell by each ear. Spring straight up and then back down, making sure to land heels-first. For additional resistance, wear ankle weights or hold a pair of dumbbells.*
2. *Leaping lunges. Get into the Forward Lunge position (see "David's Deluxe Lunge Routine" on page 66) with your hands on your hips. Leap up and switch legs in midair, landing in a lunge position.*

stiff-leg dead lift | hamstrings, glutes, erector spinae

a. Stand with your feet slightly wider than shoulder-width apart and your toes slightly turned out. (If you turn your toes slightly in, you'll work your inner hamstrings, inner glutes, and inner thighs.) Hold a pair of dumbbells against the tops of your thighs. Put your body weight in your heels, stabilize your core, and contract your shoulder blades.

b. With your body weight in your heels, inhale as you bend forward with a straight back and straight legs. Lower the dumbbells until your torso is parallel to the floor. Then focus on contracting your buttocks, pulling forward with your hips as you rise.

If your lower back bothers you during this move, concentrate on using your glutes—not your back—to lift your body. Also, make sure your body weight is in your heels. If you can't raise your big toes off the ground, your body weight isn't far enough back. Finally, remember to use your arms merely as hooks to hold the weight. You shouldn't be using your arms to hoist up the weight.

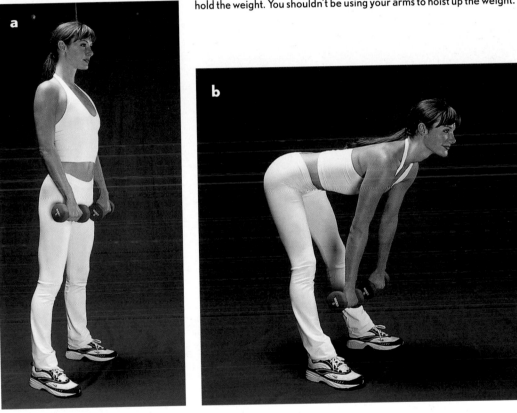

◆Distinctively David

If you have a mirror in front of you, watch yourself as you bend forward and rise. Doing so will help you keep your back flat. As you straighten, pull your pelvis forward for an extra burn in your butt. I like to tell my clients, "Give me some sex at the top of the movement." That added visualization helps them pull their hips forward, preventing them from overusing their quads.

◇ ◇ ◐ ◑ ☆

partial dead lift | lower back, glutes | ADVANCED

a. Stand with your feet slightly wider than shoulder-width apart. Hold a pair of dumbbells against the tops of your thighs. (If you're a beginner, do this with no weight first.) Focus on your heels, making sure to pull your weight into them and not into the balls of your feet. Stabilize your core and look up.

b. Focus on keeping your weight in your heels as you inhale and squat down, sticking your butt out, bending your knees, and lowering the dumbbells toward the floor with your arms extended. Keep your back flat and your abs tight through the move. Push through your heels to rise. The key is to lift and squeeze through your glutes.

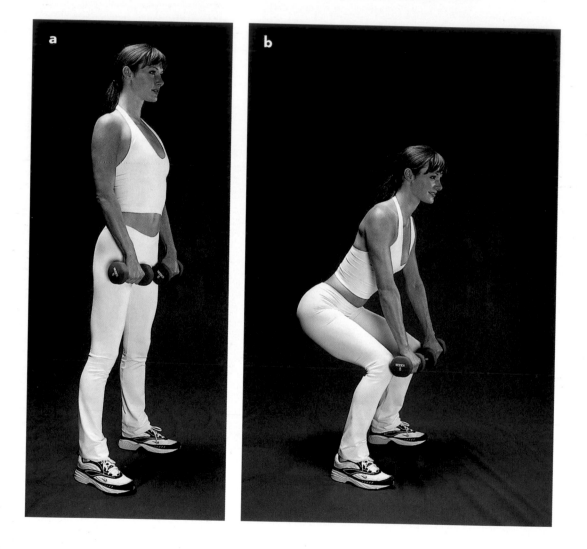

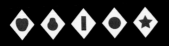

standing calf raise | gastrocnemius, soleus

Stand next to a sturdy table and lean on it for balance. (Put a book on the table and lean on that if the table is too low.) Hold a dumbbell in your other hand and keep your core stable.

Wrap one leg behind the other so that only one foot is planted on the floor. Bring your body weight forward into the ball of that foot and raise your heel off the ground as you exhale. Inhale as you slowly lower yourself to the floor.

For an extra stretch, do the move on the edge of a stair or sturdy box.

◆ Distinctively David

You can work slightly different areas of your calves simply by changing your foot position. Move your heels out to work your outer calves, and move them in to work your inner calves.

leg extension | quadriceps

Because the quadriceps play a huge role in supporting your knees, these are wonderful rehab exercises if you've had a knee injury.

a. Sit on the edge of your bench or a chair or bed while wearing ankle weights. Make sure your core is stable.

b. Exhale as you raise one leg at a time until it is extended about 80 percent (any more and you'll put too much stress on your knees). Exhale as you slowly lower your leg until your thigh forms a 90-degree angle with your calf. As you raise and lower the weight, focus on using your thighs and not your hip flexors. You should feel the movement in your lower thigh first.

If your knees hurt during this exercise, do only partial extensions in the range where you feel comfortable. When you perform leg extensions correctly, you will feel the muscles right above your knees burn first, then the burn will travel up the front of your thigh. If you feel it in your hip flexors first, you are doing it wrong. Listen to your body and modify the exercise for your needs.

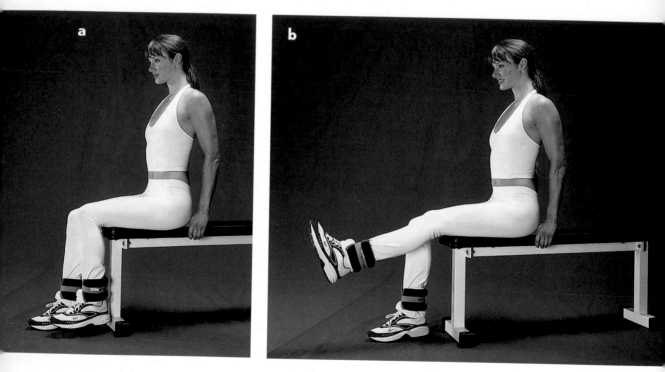

◆Distinctively David

If you are in fairly good shape, cross your arms on your chest and lean forward slightly, pushing your butt back and squeezing your glutes as you raise and lower the weight. This simple tweak will force you to isolate your quadriceps and prevent you from engaging your hip flexors.

leg curl | hamstrings

Stand while wearing a pair of ankle weights. Make sure your core is stable. You're going to be standing on one foot at a time, so lean against a sturdy table or wall if you have trouble with balance.

Exhale as you raise your right foot until your calf and thigh are bent at a 90-degree angle. You should feel the movement in your hamstrings, not in your calves. Inhale as you slowly lower your foot to the floor.

You want to focus on contracting your entire hamstring area and disengage the rest of your leg. Focus on flexing the back of your thigh as you bring your heel toward your glutes.

◆ Distinctively David

Because of the awkwardness of the movement, many people end up flexing their feet and overengaging their calves instead of their hamstrings. Instead, try to relax your calves. I find that keeping my feet pointed helps me focus on my hamstrings.

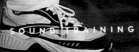

◇ ◇ ▮ ◇ ◇ ★

prone leg curl | hamstrings and adductors | ADVANCED

Wearing a pair of ankle weights, lie facedown on a decline bench (or on a flat bench if you don't have a decline bench) with your head at the top of the bench. Push your hips into the bench and exhale as you curl your calves up, squeezing through your butt and hamstrings. Inhale as your lower them to the ground. If you are strong enough, raise your thighs up off the bench at the top of the movement. That extra burn will target the roll just below your butt.

When performing leg curls, try to engage only your hamstrings. Resist the urge to power the weight up with your calves and hips. To protect your back, press your hips into the bench and remain that way throughout the movement.

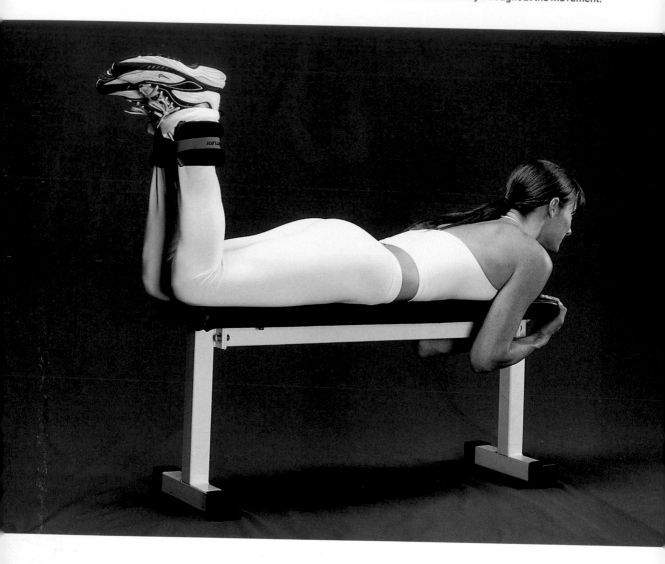

david's reverse prone scissors | glutes | ADVANCED

a. Lie facedown on your bench and spread your legs as wide as you can with your feet touching the floor.

b. Press your hips into the bench and exhale as you lift your flexed feet up and squeeze them together in one fluid movement, making sure to contract your glutes throughout the move. Squeeze your heels together at the top of the move. Inhale as you slowly lower your feet to the starting position.

   The Reverse Prone Scissors is an advanced move, and in some cases may aggravate lower-back pain. If that occurs, stop performing the exercise. The focus is on your glutes, so keep the squeeze there. Don't forget to press your hips into the bench. This will minimize the arching in your lower back.

◆Distinctively David

If you have trouble with scissors, you can train yourself to do them correctly with the following alternative exercises. At first glance, these movements may not seem taxing, but they force you to put thought into engaging the right muscle. One such exercise is the Isometric Superman, which is performed while lying facedown on a mat. There are two versions, one for beginners and one that is more advanced.

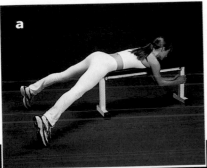

Beginners: *Lie facedown on the mat and place your hands behind your head. Lift your head and torso as high as possible and then slowly lower yourself to the floor. Focus on contracting your glutes throughout the move.*

Advanced: *Lift your head and torso, and at the same time, lift your legs while contracting your glutes. Then slowly lower yourself to the mat.*

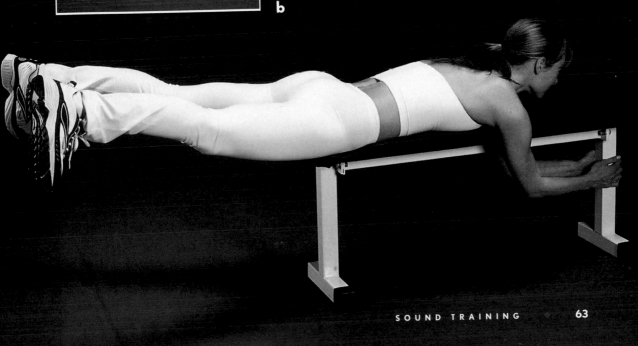

david's deluxe floor routine | adductors, glutes, abductors

a. Lie on your right side with your legs extended. Push your hips forward and contract your buttocks and abs. Exhale as you raise your left leg, pressing up through your heel with your foot flexed. (If you don't feel this move in your hips and butt, your hips are not pushed forward enough.) Inhale as you slowly lower your left leg until it's an inch above your right leg.

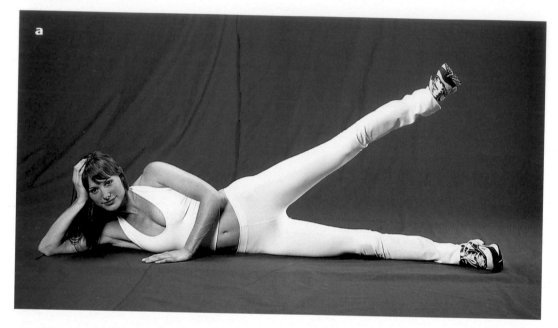

b. Without resting, inhale as you slowly pull your left knee in toward your chest, and then exhale as you extend it back so that it is just above your right leg.

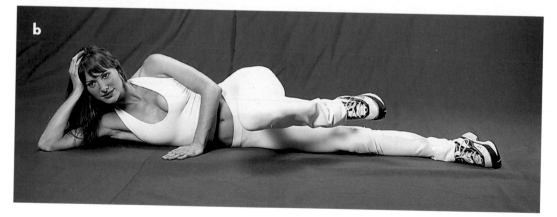

c. Inhale as you bend both of your legs into an L shape in front of your body, so that your knees are on the same plane as your hips. Put your left hand on your left buttock and push it forward. (This will force you to do the exercise correctly.) Exhale as you lift your top leg. Focus on lifting with your top knee and putting the burn in your hips and glutes. Inhale as you lower your leg.

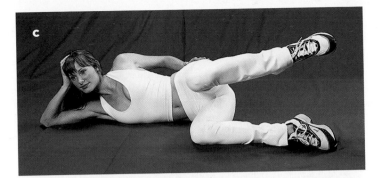

d. Exhale as you bring your thighs back in line with your torso. Bend your knees so that your calves are behind your body at a 90-degree angle to your thighs. Inhale as you lift your top leg and then lower it as you exhale.

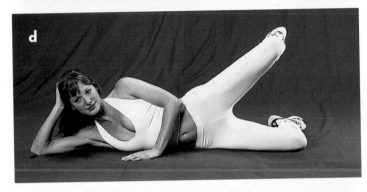

e. Inhale as you bend your left leg so that your left shin and knee are resting on the floor just in front of your extended right leg. With your hips still pushed forward and your abs contracted, exhale and raise your *right* bottom leg straight up, pressing through your heel. You should feel this in your inner thigh. Make sure your heel is pointed up and is higher than your toes.

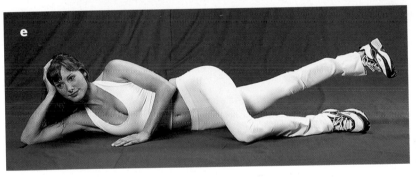

◆ Distinctively David

These moves can give you an incredibly focused burn or be a complete waste of time. Focus and visualization is key. The purpose of the Deluxe series is to engage your hips and glutes. If you're not feeling the move in your butt and outer thighs, you need to change your form and tweak the move until you get it right.

I like to do this series of moves in a giant 100- to 150-repetition set, doing all five movements one at a time over and over. By the end of the huge set, your legs will be screaming. For even more burn, I like to add pulses of each complete movement until complete muscle exhaustion.

◇ ◇ ◐ ◑ ★

david's deluxe lunge routine | hamstrings, glutes, adductors, hips

The lunge is the quintessential butt-shaping and thigh- and hip-trimming exercise, and it's been around for years. But I've added a few tweaks and twists that make them truly unique and incredibly effective. I like to perform lunges as a giant set in groups, quickly moving from one type of lunge into another. I sometimes combine them with high knee raises, kicks, squats, and even bench stepups. My lunge routine varies from day to day and from client to client, but looks something like the following routine.

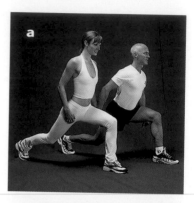

For each move, make sure you are lunging into your glutes, not your quadriceps. You should drop down after stepping out, not jut your knee forward. Your knee should never pass beyond your toes. Always keep your body weight in your heels, making sure to press up through your heels on the ascent. Once you get into each lunge position, pulse slightly up and down 15 to 20 times, focusing the weight from your heel into your glute.

a. Forward Lunge: Stand with your feet shoulder-width apart and keep your core stable. Take a large step forward with your left foot, raising the front part of your foot up as you place your heel down. (This will drive the exercise through your heel and into your glutes.) Inhale as you sink down until your thighs form right angles with your shins. Exhale as you push back up through your front heel and return to the starting position.

b. Crossover Lunge: Stand with your feet shoulder-width apart and keep your core stable. Take a large step diagonally forward with your right foot so that your foot lands at the 11 o'clock position. Plant your foot, making sure your heel hits the ground first. Inhale as you sink down until your thighs form right angles with your shins. Exhale as you push back up through your front heel and return to the starting position. Repeat with your left foot, stepping to the 1 o'clock position.

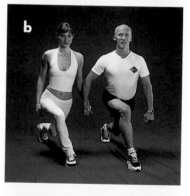

c. Reverse Lunge: Stand with your feet shoulder-width apart. Keep your core stable and your weight on your heels. Inhale as you take a large step back with your left foot, planting and then lowering your body until both legs are at right angles. Exhale as you push up through your front heel.

d. Sumo Lunge: Start in a "sumo" position with your feet slightly wider than shoulder-width apart, your knees bent, and your body weight in your heels. Take a large step sideways with your left leg, bringing your knee to your chest and then over to the left in one continuous motion. You'll resemble a sumo wrestler.

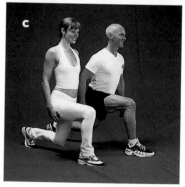

e. Asymmetrical Lunge: These lunges are difficult, but you can work up to them in three steps. Start by doing a regular Forward Lunge in place, but with the ball of your rear foot planted on a small step. Then plant the ball of your rear foot higher, such as on your bench. Finally, do them by lunging between a set of benches set 3 to 4 feet apart. This move will engage all the stabilizing muscles in your legs as well as your hip adductors.

f. The Alexandra Lunge: As you rise from any of the above lunges, rest your hands on your hips and kick your rear leg up as you move forward.

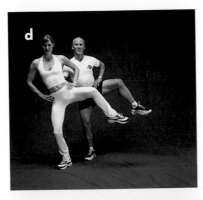

◆Try This

My lunge combinations are very effective cardio-sculpting moves, and are also constantly evolving. Here are a few:

1. *Reverse Lunges with Bench Stepups (see page 74)*
2. *Bench Stepup then step down into a Reverse Lunge*
3. *Reverse Lunge with a front high kick*
4. *Reverse Lunge with Crossover Lunge*
5. *Forward and Reverse Lunge, bringing your moving knee to your chest between lunges.*

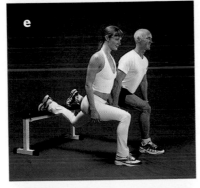

◆Try This

I'm constantly tweaking exercises into new moves and combinations, and the Side Lunge Deluxe is one of my recent favorites. You can easily turn a regular squat and a regular lunge into a side squat and side lunge by simply stepping out to the side. For the squat, start with your feet hip-width apart and step out to the right side, sinking into your right leg as you partially straighten your rear leg. For the lunge, you again step out with your right leg and sink your butt down, bending both legs equally. For both moves, rise by pushing through your right heel. I like to alternate these moves.

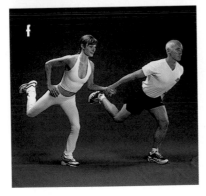

◆Distinctively David

With any of the lunge movements, do not allow your knee to go beyond your toes. If you use your heel as a guideline and an anchor, you will ensure maximum glute, hamstring, and outer thigh engagement.

If you feel the movement in your knees, you may be extending your lead knee past the safety zone (your toes). If you feel it in your rear quadriceps, you may be forgetting to bend that leg down toward the floor. While in the lunge, both legs should be bent at 90-degree angles. Throughout the move, think glutes, hamstrings, and outer thighs. Don't sway your hips.

◆ ◇ ◉ ● ◇ ✦

david's donkey deluxe | glutes, hips

a. Get on all fours with your hands under your shoulders and your knees under your hips. Make sure your back is flat, not arched or curled. Stabilize your torso by contracting your abs. Inhale as you lift your right knee off the floor and pull it straight in toward your chest.

b. Exhale as you press your right foot back and up behind you in an arcing motion. You should feel the motion in the lower part of your buttocks. Inhale as you lower your leg until your thigh is parallel to the floor.

c. Exhale as you raise your leg again, this time bent at a 90-degree angle, pulsing your heel toward the ceiling.

d. Exhale as you straighten and raise your right leg behind you. Inhale as you lower it.

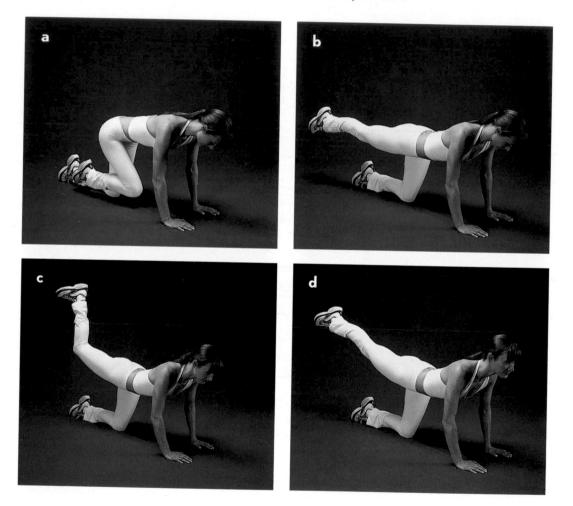

e. Exhale as you go directly into the "hydrant," bending your leg and lifting it to the side, as if you were a dog using a fire hydrant. You should feel the exercise in your buttocks and outer thigh.

◆ **Distinctively David**

I like to perform all of the Donkey movements slowly and methodically. Make sure you are contracting your glutes in every move. If you feel it in your lower back, tighten your abdomen and flatten the arch in your back. If your wrists hurt in the all-fours position, hold your hands together and rest on your forearms. Or, if you belong to a fitness club, you may have access to a donkey machine, and if you do, there is nothing better. When using the machine, go slow enough to engage just your buttocks and not your hamstrings, focusing on pressing up with your heel.

For additional intensity, you can use a pair of ankle weights. It's best to start with a lighter set (5 pounds) and increase as you are able.

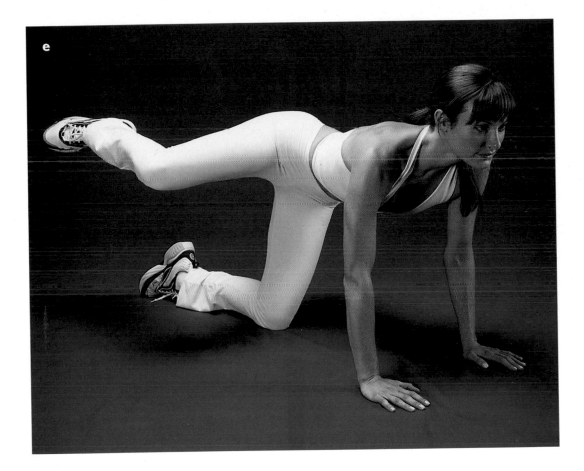

◇ ◇ ◐ ◇ ★

frog jump | hamstrings, glutes, quadriceps | ADVANCED

I've never seen a frog with a flabby butt—and this is why.

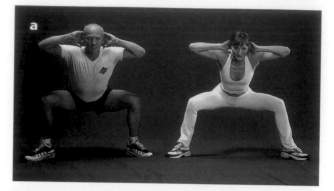

a. Squat down while sticking your butt out. Keep your knees just above—not beyond—your toes. Focus on sitting back into your heels. The power for what you will do next will come from your heels and into your glutes.

b. Spring up while thrusting your arms above your head. Land on your heels, rolling forward onto your toes. If you make the mistake of landing on your toes, you risk spraining an ankle or really messing up your knees. If you are not yet fit enough to do the jumps or you have weak ankles or a sore lower back, then simply sit way back into a squat position and hold it there for as long as you can. You can use a bar for balance, but not to hold yourself up.

Note: Do not try the Frog Jump if you have chronic back or knee problems.

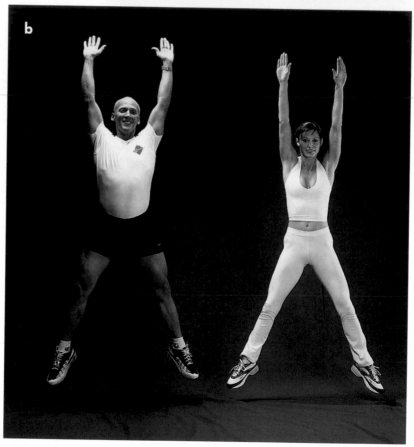

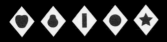

david's crab crawl | quadriceps, glutes | ADVANCED

To work both your quadriceps and your glutes, get on all fours with your butt up in the air. (Spiderman must have perfected this move as an infant.)

Put most of your weight in your legs and crawl forward with your knees slightly bent. It should look as if you are climbing a wall.

Make sure not to overextend your step, putting too much weight into your knees. Keep your core tight—and that means your abs—throughout the movement.

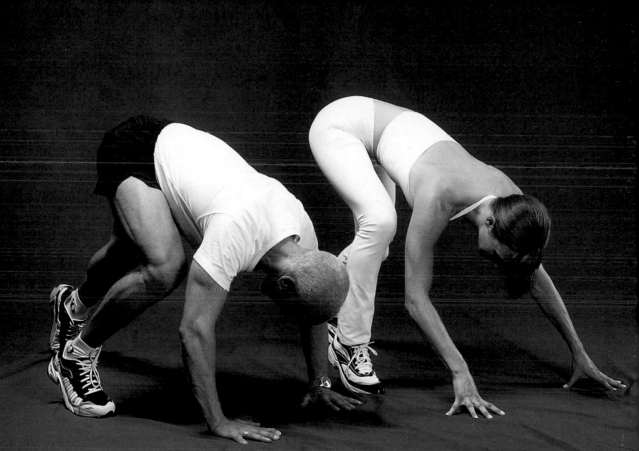

◇ ◇ ◇ ◈ ◇ ◆

david's platypus walk | glutes | ADVANCED

This is an awfully silly-looking exercise, but it will get your heart pumping and your glutes and quads burning.

Sit into a squatting position with your hands behind your head, your knees aligned with your toes, and your butt sticking back as far as you can.

Keep your core tight and walk forward while pushing off with each heel. If you perform this correctly, you'll look like a platypus—and your glutes and thighs will be on fire.

Not everyone can do the Platypus. If you have the strength and coordination to do the move, it's a great quad and glute burner. Make sure to sit back in your heels. Do not step too far forward or you'll stress your trailing knee.

◇ ◇ ◆ ◇ ◇ ★

pelvic tilt | glutes, lower rectus abdominis

a. Lie on your back on an exercise mat and place a medicine ball between your knees. If you have a large exercise ball, you can also lie on that, so that your head and shoulders are supported by the ball and your hips are off the ball.

b. Squeeze from your buttocks and exhale, curling your pelvis into a tilt. Hold for a few seconds and release.

Make sure to keep your lower back out of the movement by lifting only from your hips. The more minimal the movement, the better the contraction. Here is where "less is more" is definitely appropriate. If you are feeling it in your lower back, you are definitely engaging it more than you should be. Check to make sure your back is flat, not arched.

◆**Distinctively David**
You can press your palms into your thighs or place weights on them for a higher degree of difficulty.

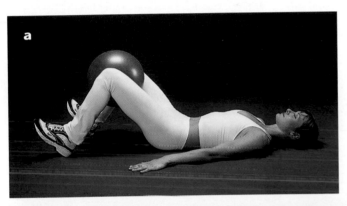

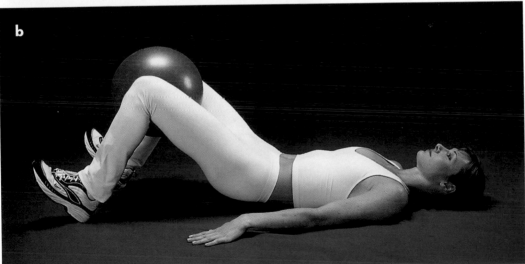

◇ ◇ ❶ ◇ ✦

bench stepup with kick and extension | glutes, quadriceps, hamstrings, gastrocnemius, soleus

a. Stand in front of a step with your core stable. Place your right foot on the step and press up through the heel of your right foot to lift your body up off the ground and onto the bench.

b. Once you've extended your right leg, bring your left knee up toward your chest. Lower yourself to the ground, switch legs, and repeat the motion on the other side.

c. Step up with your right leg again, but this time, bring your extended left leg straight behind you *without* bending your knee. Lower it and repeat on the other side.

When stepping up, it's very tempting to push off with your foot, giving yourself momentum for the step. Resist the urge, focusing on pushing instead only through the leg that is lifting your body.

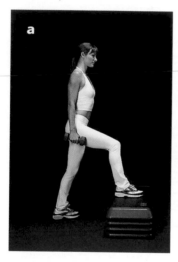

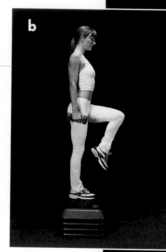

◆Distinctively David

For an additional tweak, extend both arms out and over-head as you extend your rear leg behind you. (Think Baryshnikov meets Superman.) Perform the move at a good clip, but keep the form and focus tight. Make sure not to arch your lower back.

Note: *Do not do this move if you have a history of knee or lower back problems.*

BACK

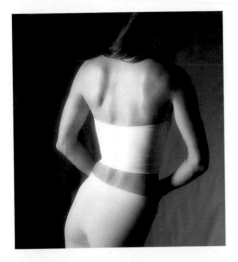

People often tell me that they have bad backs, but it's really one of the most misused medical terms going. When you have pain in your back, it usually means that you have abnormally tight hamstrings, weak abdominals, bad posture, a genetic predisposition, an actual injury, or are misusing your muscles. In other words, a bad back is often curable, as long as you pinpoint the cause.

Love those lats. After your legs, your back is the next strongest muscle group in your body. Your latissimus dorsi, or lats, run from your mid back all the way to your hips, forming a huge triangle-shaped area. Your rhomboids fill in the space between your spine and shoulder blades. And numerous smaller muscles make up the rest. Your lats form the classic V shape that you see in swimmers.

Build back strength. The stronger your entire back, the better your posture, and the less stress you place on your neck. Your latissimus dorsi and your rhomboids are both key to good posture. Lack of rhomboid strength often leads to rounded shoulders and slouching.

Stay open but don't arch. The key to working your back is core stability. Don't slouch. Keep your abs tight and *never* arch your back. When doing any pulling movement, such as a lat pull down, make sure to pull from your elbow, using your arms as hooks and bringing your shoulder blades close together. As with other exercises, retract your shoulder blades. In other words, keep your chest open and aim for your collarbone.

◇ ◇ ◉ ◇ ◇ ✦

one-arm dumbbell row | lats

a. Lean on your bench or a sturdy chair with your left knee resting on the bench and your right leg on the floor. Bend forward from the waist and rest your left hand on the bench for support. Hold a dumbbell in your right hand at your side and slightly in front of you. Make sure that your back is flat, your abs are tight, and you are focused straight ahead.

b. Exhale as you bring your right elbow straight up toward the ceiling. Keep your elbow close to your body throughout the move. At the top of the movement, pause and squeeze from your lats, making sure to keep your shoulders down. Then inhale as you slowly lower the weight, bringing it slightly forward (about 30 degrees) and turning the weight counterclockwise.

If you feel this in your shoulders, you're raising your shoulders during the movement. Keep your movement fluid, pulling from your elbow through your lats. If you feel this move in your lower back, you're arching it. Keep your abs tight.

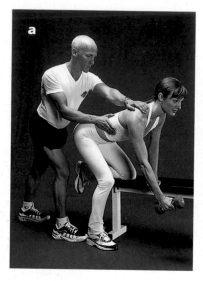

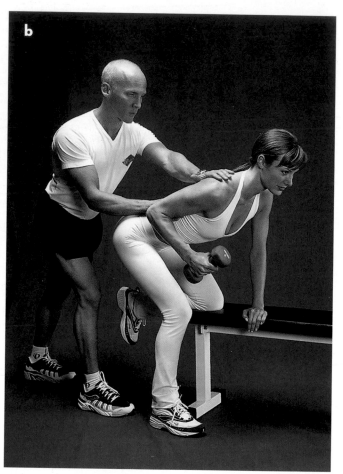

◆Distinctively David

I like to visualize that I'm starting a lawn-mower when I do this exercise. When starting a lawnmower, the choppier your movement, the more likely you'll flood the engine. It's the same here. The chop-pier you move, the less efficient the exer-cise. Pull up slo-o-owly, squeezing at the top of the movement. Take your brain and put it in your upper back.

◇ ◇ ◼ ◇ ✦

bent-over dumbbell row | lats, rhomboids, erector spinae

Stand with your feet about shoulder-width apart and bend your legs slightly so that you are sitting back on your heels. Bend forward from the waist until your torso is at a 45- to 60-degree angle. Hold a pair of dumbbells with your arms extended down, your palms facing the floor. Make sure that your back is flat, your abs are tight, and your shoulder blades are retracted. Exhale as you slowly row the dumbbells up toward your chest, keeping your elbows close to your body and squeezing your lats at the top of the movement. Inhale as you lower the weights.

To do this move correctly, you must stabilize your levator scapulae, the muscles that help properly engage your lats. Make sure to keep your abs tight and your chest open.

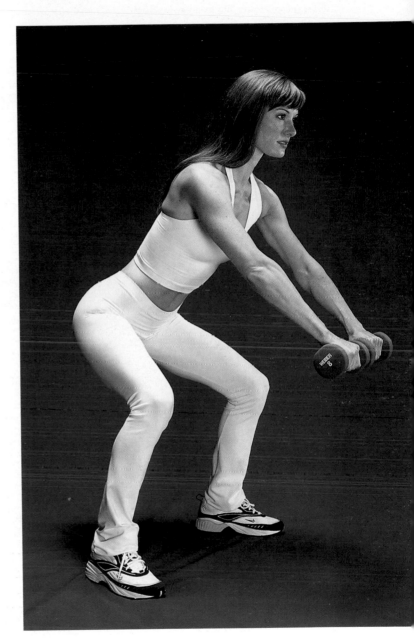

◇ ◇ ❶ ◇ ✦

under-handed dumbbell row | lower lats

To target your lower lats, try doing the Bent-Over Dumbbell Row (see page 77) with an under-handed grip. This simple tweak will create a nice line to a backless dress.

a. Hold the dumbbells with your palms facing up.

b. Pull the dumbbells in toward your body; the rest of the move is the same.
   Be careful with your form with this move. Your abs must stay tight, otherwise you will hurt your lower back. Also, focus on disengaging your biceps by pulling from your elbows and not overgripping the weight.

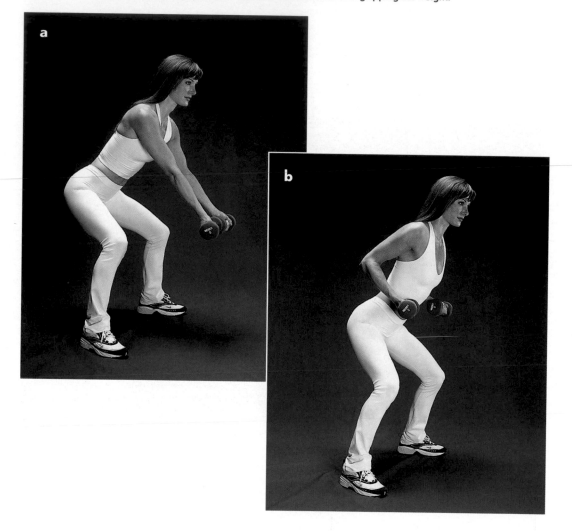

◇ ◇ ◆ ◇ ◆

pullover | upper lats, abdominals, triceps

a. Lie on your back with your head at the end of your bench. For lower-back support, bend your knees and place your feet on the bench. Hold a dumbbell with both hands from the "bell" end of the dumbbell. Straighten your arms so that your elbows are pointed toward your feet.

b. Inhale as you slowly bring the dumbbell back over and behind your head, lowering it to the line of your body. (If you're not strong enough to lower it that far, just lower it as far as you can.) Once you reach the plane of your body, exhale and raise the weight to the starting position.

Throughout the move, make sure your hips and lower back are pressed down into the bench. If you can't keep them down, have someone spot you by holding your hips down. Keep your elbows close and turned toward each other.

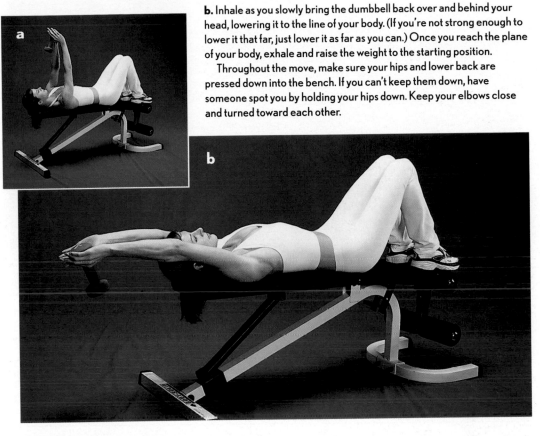

◆**Distinctively David**

Pullovers are one of the most efficient exercises around. Because you must stabilize your core, they work your back, chest, arms, and abs all at once. During the move, think about keeping your abs tight. Also, protect your shoulders by not extending the weight too far over your head and keeping your elbows pointed toward your feet.

◆Try This

I like to combine pullovers with Upright Triceps Overhead Extensions (see page 96) in a prone position. There's a nice flow to the movement, making an efficient use of my time.

a. Lie belly down on a mat with your legs extended. Place your hands behind your head. Squeeze your glutes and tighten your abs.

b. Bring your shoulders and feet off the floor as you exhale, making sure to keep your abs and glutes tight. Lengthen and press out from your fingertips and toes, as if you were lengthening your body, not just lifting up. Inhale as you lower. If the move becomes too easy, you can hold a dumbbell against the back of your head.

Note: The Superman can be a challenging isometric exercise that strengthens the lower back, abs, and glutes. It can also be a chiropractic nightmare. If you are a novice, start small by contracting and relaxing your glutes. Then contract your glutes while lifting just one leg at a time 3 to 5 inches from the floor. Then lift both legs at the same time. Finally, add your torso. Be careful not to lift too much, as this may strain your lower back.

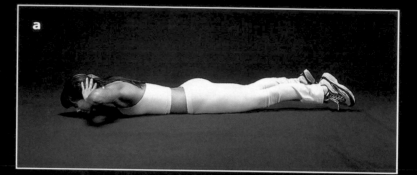

a

b

◇ ◇ ◆ ◇ ✦

good morning | erector spinae

This is an old favorite of mine that my father taught me 30 years ago. It's a perfect exercise to do to warm up your back muscles as you simultaneously tone and shape your lower back, hamstrings, glutes, and thighs. As the name implies, you can do these first thing in the morning, as soon as you get out of bed.

a. Stand with your feet slightly wider than shoulder-width apart and your hands behind your head.

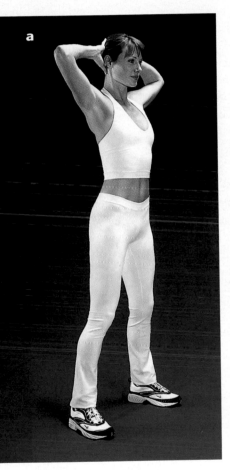

b. Bend forward from the waist, keeping your legs straight and your gaze straight ahead. Keep your back flat. Once your body is perpendicular, rise back up as your exhale. Warm up with a series of these for 30 seconds before moving onto the next phase.

Add a knee bend to the movement. Do the move as usual, but this time, once your torso is parallel to the floor, bend your knees and lower your butt toward the floor, finishing the movement by straightening your legs and standing up at the same time. The second part of the move—the knee bend—must be done slowly and carefully. Make sure to engage your glutes throughout the move by sticking your butt out as much as possible. That will take the pressure off your knees.

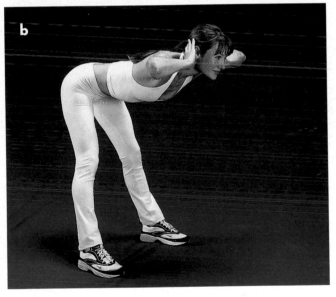

◆Distinctively David

The Good Morning is a basic lower-back warmup that can be used at all levels. At the beginner level, concentrate on getting the form down and focusing on stretching out your lower back and hamstrings. As your level of proficiency improves, you can add weight by placing a pair of light dumbbells behind your head.

SHOULDERS

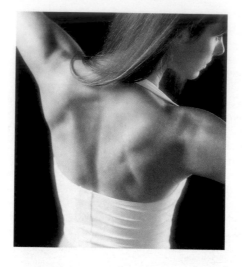

I like to say that two of the things God created on the 6th day—before he decided that he needed to rest—were shoulders and knees, the two most injured joints in the body.

Shoulders are particularly vulnerable because there are so many ways to mess them up. Your largest shoulder muscle is called your deltoid, which actually forms the bulk of what most people think of as their shoulder. The muscle that runs from your shoulder to your lower neck is your trapezius. But what most people injure is one of a series of small muscles around the shoulder blade collectively known as the rotator cuff.

The shoulder exercises I recommend are basic—presses, various lateral movements, and front raises—but they are also the most effective ones for building shoulder strength. You must, however, do them correctly.

Elbow first. During all shoulder movements, lead with your elbow. Take a minute right now and raise your arm to the side of your body, bringing your thumb up first. Then raise your arm, but lead with your elbow. Feel the difference? The latter is the way you want to feel during every shoulder exercise. It works your deltoids in a more specific and controlled way.

Other than leading with your elbow, these exercises require you to use good posture, with your shoulder blades retracted and your core stable.

Don't forget to warm up. Before doing any shoulder exercises, warm up with light weights doing the same movements that the exercise entails. Or, warm up with a series of jumping jacks or shoulder rotations— anything to get your shoulder area nice and warm. And don't forget to finish up with some stretches. (See "David's Stretches" on page 40.)

◇ ◇ ◆ ◇ ◆ ★

military/shoulder press | deltoids, triceps

a. Sit on the end of an adjustable bench with the back of the bench set at a 90-degree angle. Firmly press your buttocks and back against the seat back and make sure your abs are tight. Hold a pair of dumbbells above your shoulders either with your palms facing each other in a neutral grip or with your palms facing forward, making sure your shoulder blades are retracted and your chest is open. Stabilize your torso by firming your abdominal muscles.

b. Exhale as you press the dumbbells straight up above your shoulders. Extend your arms, but stop before your elbows lock. Inhale as you lower the dumbbells to the starting position.

If you feel pain in your neck, you are probably rounding your shoulders or engaging your trapezius muscles too much.

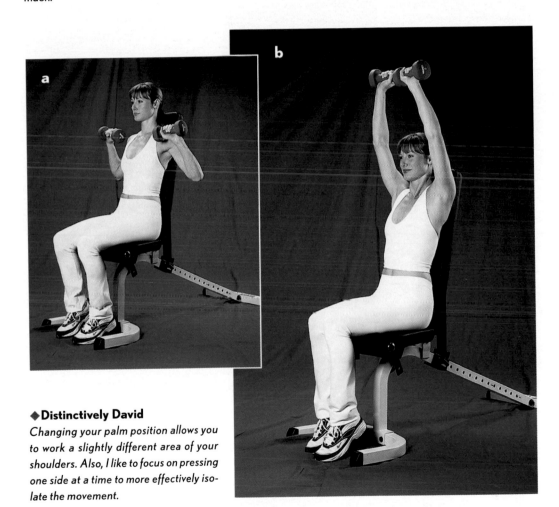

◆Distinctively David
Changing your palm position allows you to work a slightly different area of your shoulders. Also, I like to focus on pressing one side at a time to more effectively isolate the movement.

◇ ○ ◐ ● ◇ ✦

side lateral | side deltoids

a. Stand with your torso stable and your feet shoulder-width apart. Hold a pair of dumbbells at your sides. Concentrate on keeping your abs tight and your shoulder blades retracted.

b. Raise your arms out to the sides, focusing on raising your elbows and pinkies first. Make sure your palms face the floor, not forward. When using the correct form, you will feel your side deltoids burning.

If you have trouble keeping the correct palm position, the weight is probably too heavy. This move is not about a lot of weight, it's about good form.

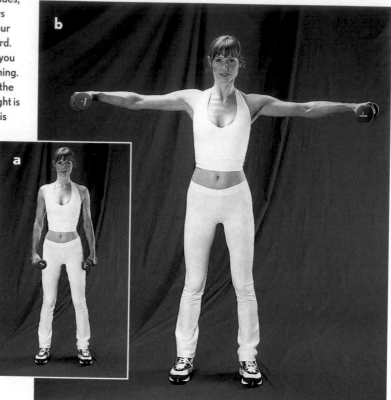

◆Distinctively David
If you have something steady to hold on to, lean one hand on the object so that you can perform one-arm Side Laterals without moving your torso.

◆Try This—Proceed with Caution

If you've had a serious shoulder injury, many shoulder movements are contraindicated, but there are a few that are still appropriate:

◆ *Modified Side Lateral. Bend your arms at a 90-degree angle and use a very light weight. You'll somewhat resemble the "funky chicken."*
◆ *Manual-Resistance Side Lateral. Hold your arms out in the side lateral position with no weight. Keep them there as long as possible while pulsing up and down slightly.*

◆ ◆ **◆** ◆ ★

front raise | front deltoids

a. Stand with your torso stable and your feet shoulder-width apart. Hold a pair of dumbbells held just in front of your thighs. Concentrate on keeping your abs tight and your shoulder blades retracted.

b. Exhale as you lift your arms forward and slightly in toward the center of your body, making sure to lead with your elbows. As you raise the weight, turn your palms down and finish with your arms parallel with the floor. Inhale as you lower the weights.

For an additional tweak, turn the dumbbells slightly down at the top of the movement, as if you were pouring two glasses of milk. To work your inner deltoid a bit more, try doing the Front Raise with a hammer grip so that your palms are facing one another and you are leading with your thumbs.

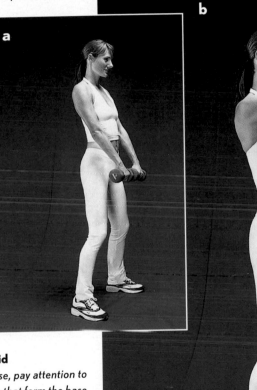

◆**Distinctively David**

Throughout the exercise, pay attention to your traps, the muscles that form the base of your neck. Are they tense? If so, you're not doing the exercise correctly. Try to relax your neck muscles. If you can't, the weight is too heavy.

◇ ◇ ◑ ◇ ✦

david's press | anterior deltoid | ADVANCED

a. Stand or sit on a bench with your butt and abs tight. Hold a pair of dumbbells at about chin level with your palms facing you.

b. Exhale as you press the dumbbells up. Inhale as you slowly lower the weights back to the starting position, making sure to keep your abs tight and stable. Make sure your elbows stay close to your body throughout the movement.

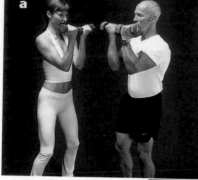

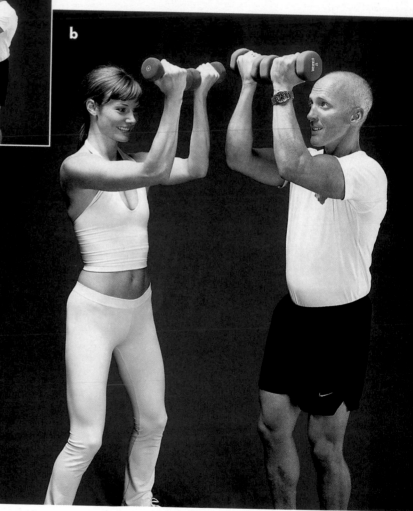

◆**Distinctively David**

If you listen to your body, it will tell you when to stop or skip an exercise. I don't believe in the saying, "No pain, no gain." You should never feel pain. Instead, I like to say, "No maximum effort, no gain." Steady pain does not lead to gain, but rather to injury.

◇ ◇ ◆ ◆ ◇ ◈

shrug | trapezius

This is a great rehab exercise for people with neck problems because the traps support the neck.

a. Stand or sit on the end of a bench, keeping your abs tight and your back flat. Retract your shoulder blades and hold a pair of dumbbells at your sides.

b. Exhale as you shrug your shoulders straight up. As you shrug, visualize your trapezius muscles contracting. Inhale as you lower the weight, letting your shoulders relax, and feeling the stretch through your neck and shoulders.

It is really important to keep your neck relaxed throughout the movement and to focus on primarily using your trapezius muscles to lift the weight.

◆**Distinctively David**

Focus on lifting through your traps—not with your arms. Even though shoulder shrugs are important, especially if you have neck problems, I don't put too much emphasis on them in my core program. If you shrug too much weight, you'll overdevelop your traps and end up looking simian.

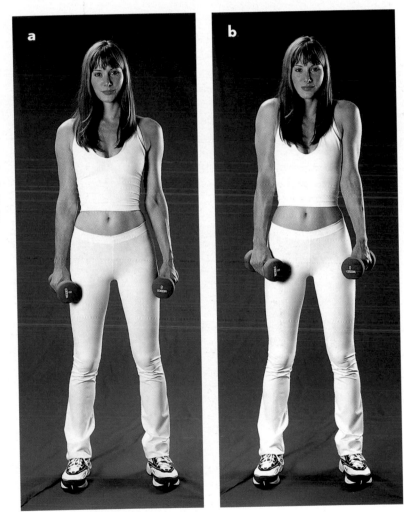

◇ ◇ ◉ ◇ ✦

david's "the chicken" | deltoids

I often give this move to clients who are rehabilitating a rotator cuff injury and can't perform core shoulder exercises such as the Side Lateral (see page 84).

a. Stand with your torso stable and your feet shoulder-width apart. Hold a dumbbell in each hand at chest level with your elbows at your sides.

b. Slowly rotate your elbows up, as if you were a chicken flapping its wings, except perform these much slower than a chicken would.

Make sure to lead from your elbows, focusing on your side deltoids.

◆Try This

I like to combine Chickens with partial Front Raises (see page 85). These two exercises will really get the shoulders warmed up and ready to go. I also like to do them at the end of a huge drop set of shoulder exercises. Once you can't do another Side Lateral (see page 84), switch to the Chicken. I also like to mix in jumping jacks and Shadowboxing (page 112) with dumbbells for 30 seconds to 1 minute for a great cardio-sculpting blast.

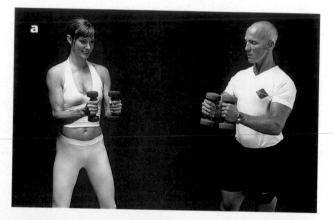

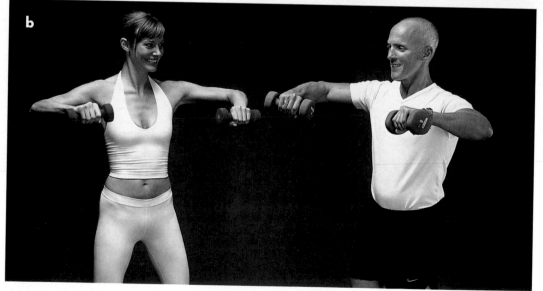

ARMS

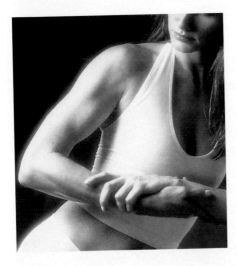

For my newer clients who are pressed for time, I often omit specific arm exercises. That's because you can work your biceps, the muscle on the front top of your arm, when you work your back during any pulling motion. And you can work your triceps, the muscle on the top back of your arm, when you work your chest, during any pressing movement. So, if time is an issue, you may be able to get by without specific isolation exercises for your arms.

On the other hand, if you want true definition, you must isolate your arm muscles. Your biceps and triceps are not as strong as your shoulders or back, so you must take those larger muscles out of the picture when working your arms. That means not throwing your elbows and shoulders forward or using momentum to raise your dumbbells. Instead, you must focus on keeping your elbows close to your body with your wrists locked.

Relax with the mind-body connection. Your biceps and triceps are antagonists (opposite muscles), meaning that when one contracts, the other relaxes, or at least it should. When doing any biceps exercise, use your mind-body connection to make sure your triceps are relaxed, and vice versa.

Develop beauty and brawn. Many people, myself included, refer to the biceps as the beauty and the triceps as the brawn. For beautiful arms, you need to develop your biceps. For more strength in pressing movements (such as the bench press) and to prevent "arm jiggle" when you shake someone's hand or wave hello or goodbye, you need to focus on your triceps.

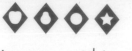

biceps curl | biceps

a. Stand with your feet shoulder-width apart and hold a pair of dumbbells near your hips with your palms facing forward. Make sure that your torso is stable and your shoulder blades are retracted. Keep your elbows at your sides and pulled back so as not to engage your shoulders.

b. Exhale as you curl the dumbbells toward your chest, making sure to keep your elbows close to your body and your shoulders as motionless as possible. Put your brain into your biceps, concentrating on using only those muscles to lift the weight, and simultaneously relaxing your triceps and shoulders. Inhale as you slowly lower the weight to the starting position.

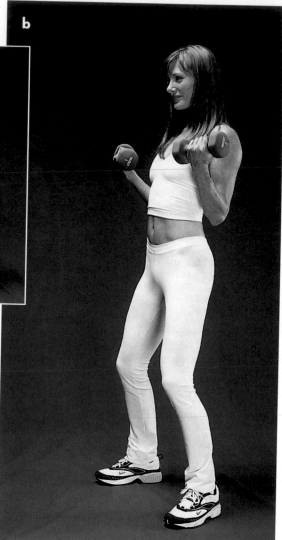

If you have lower-back problems, do the move while sitting on your bench rather than standing. A perfectly performed curl will generally go three-quarters of the way up the arm. In other words, disengaging the shoulders will result in a tighter, smaller biceps movement.

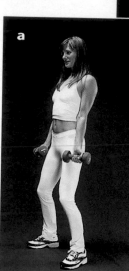

◆Distinctively David

Vary the section of your biceps that you work by curling your dumbbells with your palms forward, with your palms facing in, or starting with your palms facing in and then rotating at the top. You can also bring your hands slightly further away from your body—with your elbows still against your sides—to work a slightly different area of your biceps.

◇ ◇ ▮ ◇ ✦

forearm raise | extensors

a. Sit on your bench, bend from the waist, and hold a dumbbell in your right hand just beyond the edge of the bench with your palm facing up and your left arm resting on your left thigh.

b. Using your wrists, raise the dumbbells so that your knuckles come toward your forearm. Only your hand and wrist should move. Lower the dumbbell to the starting position.

c. After completing enough repetitions to fatigue your forearm, switch your grip so that your palm faces the floor. Again, curl the dumbbell using your wrist, this time bringing the back of your hand toward your arm.

This move is about your forearms. Make sure the rest of your arm is fully relaxed. Pay careful attention to not overextending your hand in either direction.

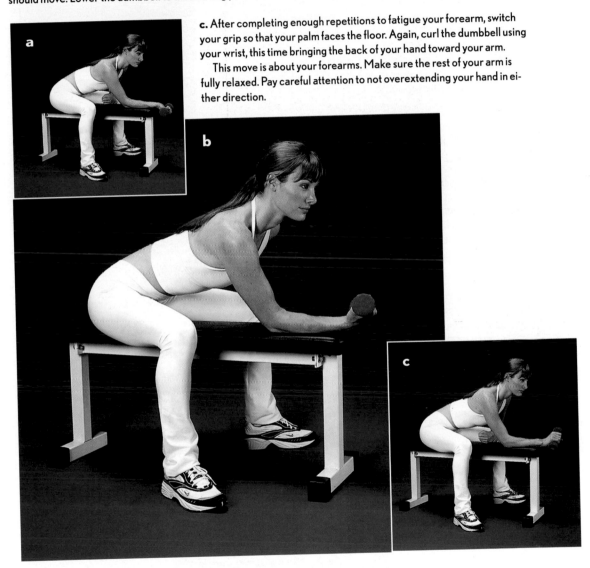

incline biceps curl | biceps

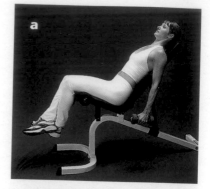

a. Adjust your bench to a 75-degree angle and sit into it so that your back and hips are firmly resting on the seat back. If your feet don't touch the ground, cross your ankles. Hold a pair of dumbbells at your sides with your arms extended.

b. Exhale as you slowly curl one arm up at a time, making sure to keep your elbows as close to your sides as you can with the dumbbells turned out slightly. (If the dumbbell hits the bench or your hips, angle your hands out even more, still keeping your elbows close to the bench.) Inhale as you lower the dumbbells to the starting position.

Throughout the move, make sure to keep your shoulders motionless and your shoulder blades retracted.

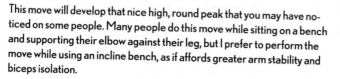

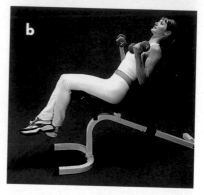

concentration curl | biceps peak

This move will develop that nice high, round peak that you may have noticed on some people. Many people do this move while sitting on a bench and supporting their elbow against their leg, but I prefer to perform the move while using an incline bench, as if affords greater arm stability and biceps isolation.

a. Adjust your bench to a 75-degree angle and stand sideways behind it, resting the back of your left arm on the bench. Hold a dumbbell in your left hand and put your right hand behind your back.

b. Exhale as you slowly curl your left hand toward your upper arm, keeping your left shoulder motionless. At the top of the move, pause and squeeze your left biceps. Inhale as you slowly lower your arm back to the starting position.

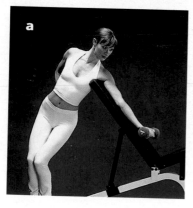

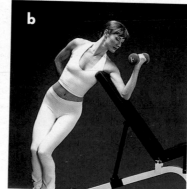

◆**Distinctively David**

If you have trouble keeping your shoulder stable, rest your right arm on your left shoulder to hold it in place. If that doesn't help, reduce the amount of weight you are lifting. This move is about fully extending your arm to get the entire muscle engaged, and about squeezing your biceps at the top, not about how much weight you can lift.

◇ ◇ ◇ ◆

hammer curl | outer biceps

Simply changing your palm position will work a slightly different area of your biceps.

a. Stand with your feet shoulder-width apart. Hold a pair of dumbbells at your sides with your palms facing in.

b. Exhale as you curl the dumbbells up, keeping your elbows close to your sides.

If you feel the curls in your shoulders, you are probably rounding them forward. Pull your shoulders down and retract your shoulder blades, keeping your chest open. Pull your elbows back. Resist the urge to swing the weight up with your back and hips.

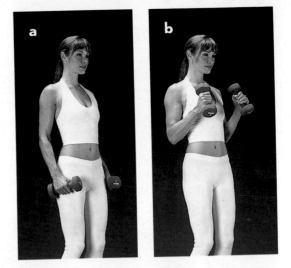

◆Try This

Many men like to sculpt large, well-rounded biceps. To do so, you must work your biceps from all directions. That means doing multiple moves that target different aspects of the biceps muscles. One of my favorite combination moves addresses two sections of the biceps simultaneously. Start curling up as a Hammer Curl and then, just before the top, turn your palms up into a regular Biceps Curl (see page 90). This exercise is just as effective for women because it shapes and sculpts the biceps completely. Women may want to use a slightly lighter weight.

◇ ◇ ◇ ◆

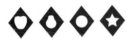

reverse-grip curl | extensors

Stand with your feet shoulder-width apart while holding a pair of dumbbells at your waist. Grasp the dumbbells so that your palms are facing your thighs. Make sure your torso is stable, and that your shoulder blades are pulled down and close together. Exhale as you curl the dumbbells toward your chest, making sure to keep your elbows close to your body and your shoulders as motionless as possible. Inhale as you slowly lower the weights to the starting position.

Note: This move is similar to the Biceps Curl (see page 90), except you are reversing your grip.

As with the Biceps Curl, be sure to disengage the rest of your body when doing this move. Slowly curl the weight up, and slowly release it. You don't need a lot of weight to make this one effective.

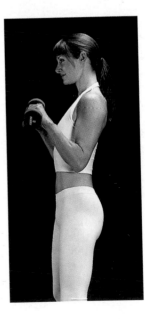

◆ ◇ ◇ ✦

skull crusher | triceps

a. Lie on your back on your bench and hold a pair of dumbbells extended above your chest with your hands slightly narrower than shoulder-width apart. Make sure your elbows are pointing forward and are as close together as possible.

b. While keeping your upper arms stable, inhale as you slowly bend your arms from the elbows, lowering the dumbbells toward either side of your forehead (thus the name Skull Crusher). Exhale as you slowly raise the weights in an arc—up and slightly away from you—to the starting position.

   Throughout the move, focus on moving only the part of your arm between your elbows and fingers. If you feel this move in your shoulders, you're not pressing your shoulders back enough against the bench. If you feel it in your elbows, you're locking out too much at the top of the movement.

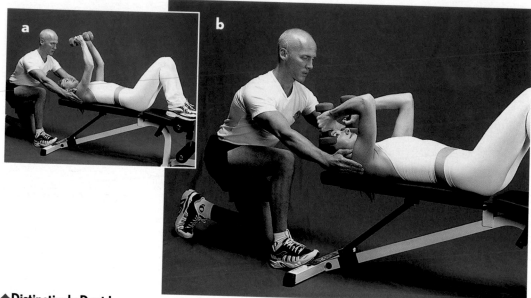

◆ **Distinctively David**

Your wrist position is important for Skull Crushers, but the right position varies from person to person. You want your wrists locked in a position that allows you to focus on your triceps. As you do the exercise, use your mind to feel out the most effective wrist position for you, and then lock into it.

◆ Try This

I like to superset Skull Crushers with bench presses that target the triceps. When targeting the triceps with a bench press, keep your elbows close to your body and the dumbbells fairly close together. I like to add one more move that is guaranteed to make your triceps sing. It involves doing a similar move to a Skull Crusher, but turning the dumbbell so that you bring it down to the opposite side of your chest rather than your skull. I can hear them singing already.

◇ ◇ ◇ ✦

triceps kickback | triceps

a. While holding a dumbbell at your side, go into a lunge stance and bend forward from the waist, making sure to keep your back straight. Bend your elbow and hold the weight so that your palm is facing forward. Rest your other hand on your thigh.

b. Exhale as you press your hand back, straightening your arm, making sure to keep your wrist locked.

c. Rotate your wrist so that your palm ends up facing behind you.
 Keep your elbows close to your body throughout the move and concentrate on keeping your shoulders and upper arms motionless. If you feel this move in your lower back, your abs are not tight enough.

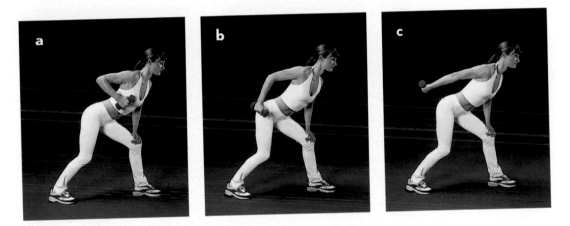

◆Distinctively David
I love to switch hand positions on triceps exercises. For one, it keeps me from getting bored. Second, it makes my work-outs more effective. Simply switching your grip or using a different type of weight can work your muscle in new ways, giving you better definition.

◆Try This
I like to combine Triceps Kickbacks with Reverse-Grip Pushups (see page 99) against a bar or on the floor, and some-times even follow up with David's Reverse Crab (see page 98) for a crazy, giant set of triceps-burning exercises. Sometimes I swap Reverse-Grip Pushups for Close-Grip Pushups (see "Try This" on page 46) with my fingers pointing in and toward one another.

◇ ◇ ◇ ✦

upright triceps overhead extension | triceps

a. Stand with your feet shoulder-width apart with a dumbbell in your right hand and your torso stable. Raise your arm so that your right arm is extended and your right bicep is near your head. Make sure your shoulder blades are retracted, expanding your chest. Keep your abs tight.

b. Inhale as you slowly bend your elbow so that the dumbbell drops behind your head. Try to get a nice, full triceps stretch at the bottom of the movement. Then exhale as you slowly press the dumbbell back up, making sure to move from your elbow, keeping your upper arm motionless.

If your back hurts during this move, you are probably arching it. Be sure to keep your abs tight throughout the move.

◆**Distinctively David**
Some people do this exercise by clasping one dumbbell with both hands and lowering it behind their heads. But I like to work one arm at a time because it gives me an even workout on both sides.

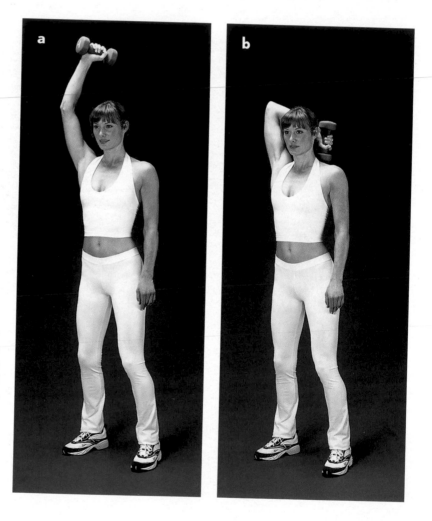

◆ ◆ ◆ ★

dips on a bench | triceps

If you have shoulder problems, skip this exercise.

a. Sit with your buttocks on the edge of your bench. Place your palms on the bench on either side of your butt, and then scoot your butt off the bench so that you are balanced on your hands.

b. Inhale as you slowly bend your elbows and lower your body, keeping your body as close to the bench as you can, and your elbows close to your body. Stop once your arms are bent at 90-degree angles. Exhale and use your triceps to push yourself back up.

Keep your shoulder blades retracted and close together throughout this move. If you slouch, you'll be working your traps more than your triceps. If you feel this move in your shoulders, your elbows probably are not close enough together.

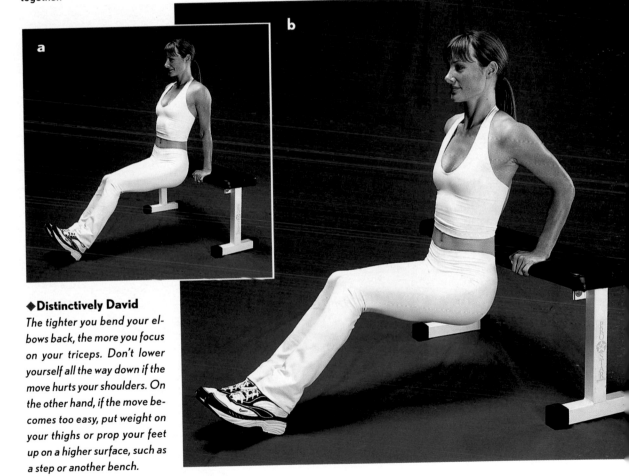

◆Distinctively David
The tighter you bend your elbows back, the more you focus on your triceps. Don't lower yourself all the way down if the move hurts your shoulders. On the other hand, if the move becomes too easy, put weight on your thighs or prop your feet up on a higher surface, such as a step or another bench.

◇ ◇ ◇ ✦

david's reverse crab | triceps | ADVANCED

a. Sit on a mat with your hands behind your butt with your fingers pointing forward and your knees bent.

b. Press through your triceps to lift your butt off the floor.

c. Walk backward on your hands and feet. You should feel your triceps screaming. Alternate these with pushups for a truly deluxe burn.
   To do this exercise correctly, you must use the same form as for all triceps work: Keep your shoulders back, don't lock your elbows, keep your abs tight, and don't arch your lower back.

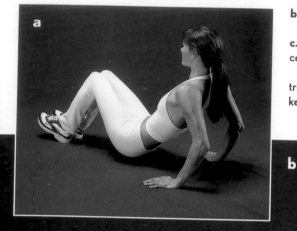

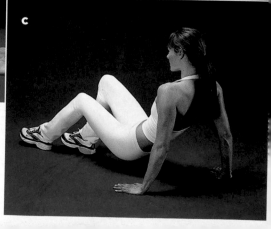

◆ ◆ ◆ ✦

reverse-grip pushup | triceps | ADVANCED

This twist on the Standard Pushup (see page 45) will target your triceps and lower chest.

a. Lean against the side edge of your bench, a bar, or the back of a sturdy chair. Reverse your grip so that your knuckles are facing you.

b. Bring your elbows in close to your body and inhale as you lower yourself, exhaling as you press up through your triceps. The main differences between this and the Standard Pushup are your arm position and your focus. For this move, your elbows are drawn against your sides, and you're focusing on your triceps, not your chest.

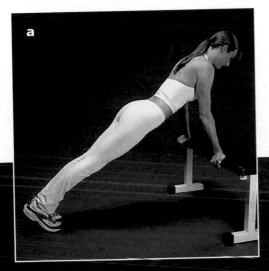

◆Try This

I like to combine Triceps Kickbacks (see page 95) with Reverse-Grip Pushups and Close-Grip Pushups (see "Try This" on page 46). To change a Close-Grip Pushup from a chest to a triceps exercise, simply bring your elbows in close to your body and put your brain into your triceps. This focus will allow you to develop upper arms that stand still in the strongest wind.

ABDOMINALS

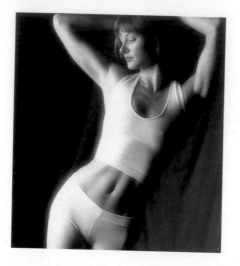

Your abdominals provide you with balance and stability, and you should be using them when you do every single exercise and even just when sitting at your desk or walking to the store. Throughout the day, be aware of when you slouch. Keep your abs tight by sucking in your belly.

Your abdominals are made up of four large muscles. Your transverse abdominis is the deepest of these four muscles. You use this muscle when you pull in your belly. Your internal oblique and external oblique muscles form the sides of your abdomen and allow you to twist from side to side. Your rectus abdominis makes up the front of your abs, running from your pubic bone to your lower ribs. This muscle is the main player when you do a crunch, the quintessential ab-strengthening exercise.

Crunch it right. Give me 25 perfect crunches so that your abs are screaming, rather than 50 crunches with bad form. For all types of crunches, press your lower back into the floor and squeeze your buttocks. That will keep your body stable.

Make it a fluid move. Fixate on a spot above your head to keep your neck open with your eyes and chin facing up. Done correctly, a crunch should feel fluid. Move slowly with your breath, contracting your abs throughout the movement.

Feel the move. When you work your lower abdominal area, be sure to engage your lower abs and not your hip flexors. The most common mistake people make is just lifting their thighs up and pulling them into their chest, which works mostly their thighs and hip flexors rather than their abs. Lift from your hips and roll your hips up or toward your chest. When done correctly, you'll feel it in your lower abs from behind your belly button downward.

◆ ◐ ◑ ◆ ★

basic crunch | rectus abdominis

Lie on your back on a mat on the floor with your legs bent and your feet flat on the mat. Place both hands as far down your upper back as possible, so that your head is resting on your forearms. (I developed this position for supermodel James King, who often complained of neck pain during her crunches.) Visualize gravity pulling your belly button to the floor, flattening your back. If you have trouble keeping your back flat against the floor, lift your hips and then lower your back down first, then your buttocks. Your buttocks may be slightly in the air. That's okay as long as your back is flat. (You can also try placing your feet against a stable surface.)

Focus on your abs as you simultaneously relax your back, neck, shoulders, and arms. Breathe out as you crunch up, starting from your lower belly and curling one vertebra at a time until you reach your shoulders. Lift from your shoulders, making sure not to use your hands or arms to yank your head off the ground. Once you can curl up no farther, slowly lower your body. Go directly into your next repetition before your shoulders reach the floor to keep a constant contraction in your abs.

Throughout the move, keep your gaze straight up toward the ceiling. That will keep your face, neck, and arms relaxed as well as prevent you from using your hands to jerk your head forward.

◆ **Distinctively David**

If you have lower-back problems, rest your legs on a large rubber or medicine ball. It will keep your back in position and will prevent you from using your hip flexors.

◇ ◇ ◐ ◑ ◇ ◇ ☆

oblique crunch | external and internal obliques

a. Get into the Basic Crunch position (see page 101) and rest your right foot on your left knee.

b. Exhale as you bring your left elbow toward your right knee. Your knee should remain in place; don't bring your knee to your elbow. Slowly lower yourself, stopping before your shoulders rest on the floor, and repeat.
    During the move, make sure you are lifting with your abdominal muscles and not with your arms or back. If your neck hurts, relax your grip and focus on keeping your elbows open and your opposite shoulder lifting to the opposite knee.

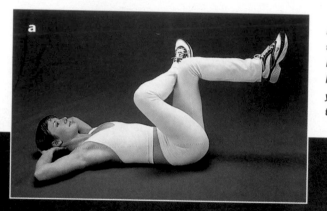

◆ Distinctively David
Many people rest between crunches, lowering their back, shoulders, and head to the ground. But you can get more results in less time if you keep your abs contracted the entire time. Lower your body, but stop before your shoulders come to the ground.

◇ ◇ ◈ ◇ ◇

reverse crunch | lower rectus abdominis

a. Lie on your back on a mat and hold a large rubber ball between your legs. This will force you to keep your back in position and to isolate your lower abs. Place your hands under your buttocks.

b. Bring your legs up so that your feet are facing the ceiling and your thighs are close to your belly. Exhale as you simultaneously pull your belly button down into the mat and roll up from your hips, concentrating on scooping out your lower abs.

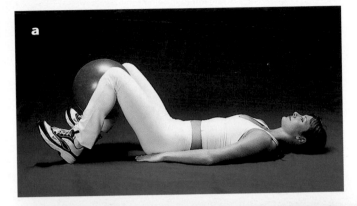

a

You should feel the movement in your lower abs first, not in your hip flexors. Take your brain and stick it into your belly button, sucking it in to contract your lower abdominal muscles.

◆**Distinctively David**

To make this move harder, use a weighted medicine ball between your knees. Or, bring your legs straight up at a right angle to your torso. In this perpendicular position, take extra precaution to protect your lower back. Concentrate on lifting from your hips and pressing your heels into the air.

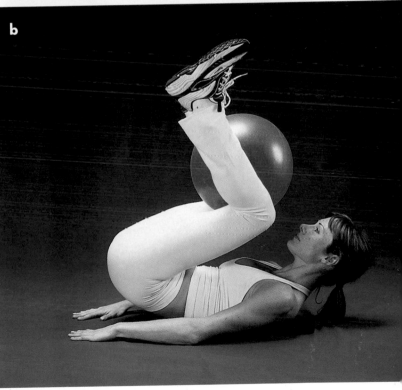

b

◆Try This

When I'm crunched for time, I sometimes like to combine a Basic Crunch (see page 101) and a Reverse Crunch into one move called a Double Crunch. Just be sure not to jerk your head off the floor with your hands or use momentum to rock your hips up. I also do what I call Abs Deluxe, where I alternate the Basic Crunch with the Reverse Crunch.

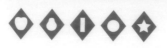

african dance step | external and internal obliques

Stand with your hands behind your head and your elbows in line with your ears. Simultaneously lift your left knee up and out to the side and lower your left elbow to meet it. Repeat on the other side. Alternate sides until your obliques are burning.

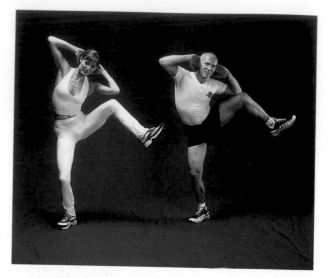

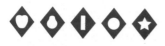

oblique twist | external and internal obliques

a. Lie on a mat on your back and turn your legs so that they form an "L" to the left side of your body. Bend your knees into a 90-degree angle. Cradle your head in your hands.

b. Exhale as you crunch up, making sure not to jerk your head up with your hands. If this is easy, do a double crunch by lifting your legs and upper body toward each other at the same time.

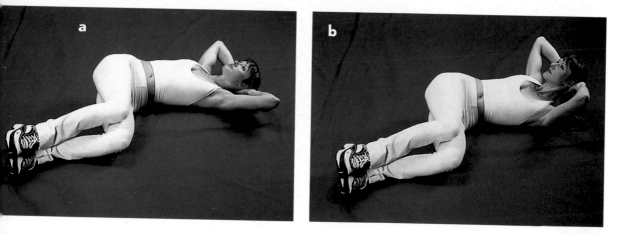

torso turn | external and internal obliques

a. Stand with your feet hip-width apart and your hands behind your head. Stabilize your core by tightening your abs.

b. Twist from side to side, making sure not to pinch your lower back by overtwisting. The movement should be slow and controlled, not jerky.

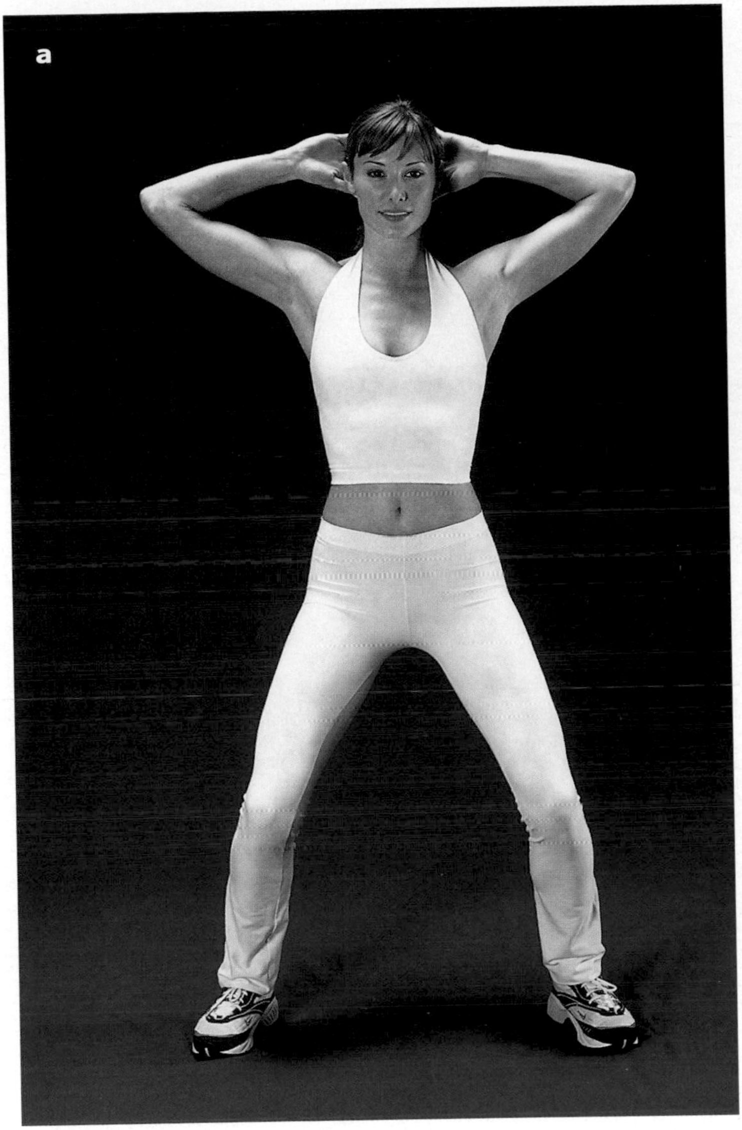

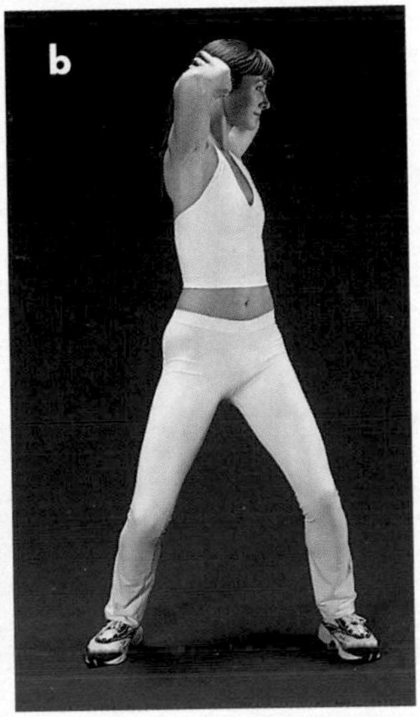

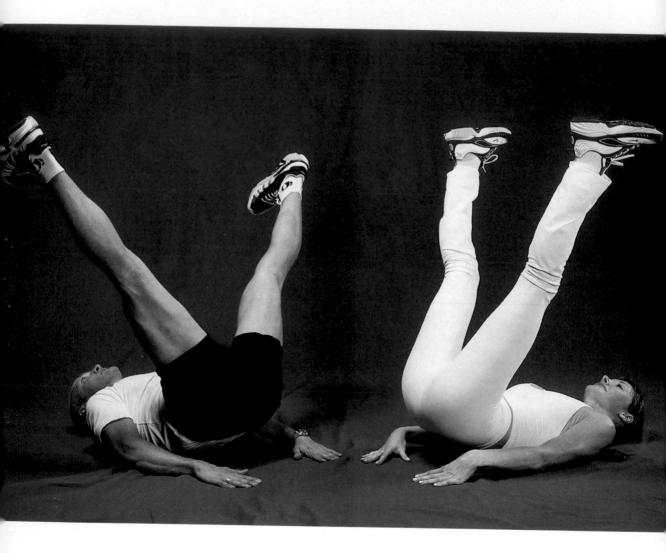

scissors reverse crunch | lower rectus abdominis

Lie on your back on a mat. Bring both legs into the air so that your legs form a 90-degree angle with your body. Stabilize your core and make sure your abs are tight. Bring your feet apart so your legs form a scissor shape, and then pull from your hips into a Reverse Crunch (see page 103). Make sure your feet are flexed. If the move becomes too easy, use 5- to 10-pound ankle weights or ask a friend or your trainer to apply gentle pressure downward to your ankles.

If your lower back hurts during this move, limit your range of motion and be sure to disengage your hip flexors. Additionally, be sure to tighten up your abs and keep them contracted throughout the movement.

◆ ◇ ◆ ❙ ◆ ✦

leg circles | lower rectus abdominis | ADVANCED

a. Sit on a mat with your hands behind your butt and your fingers pointing forward. Your legs should be bent and raised in front of you.

b. Making sure to keep your ankles together, slowly draw circles with your feet, going both clockwise and counter-clockwise.

◆Distinctively David

If you have any problems with your lower back, please avoid this exercise.

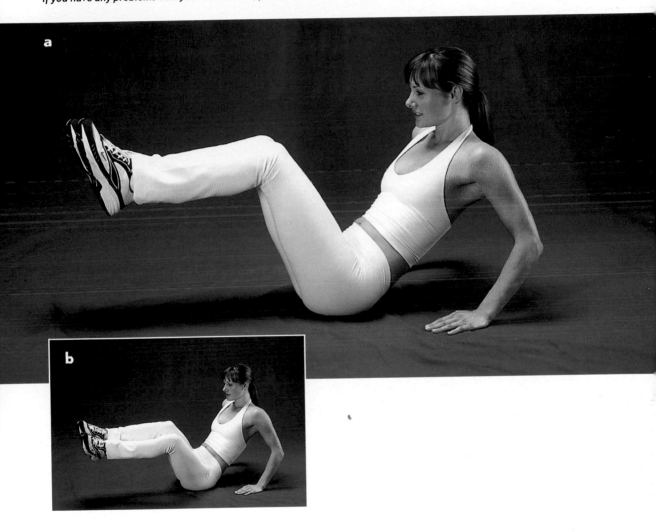

◇ ◇ ◗ ◗ ◇ ✪

david's isometric ab | lower rectus abdominis | ADVANCED

I started this move while running a boot camp on the beach in the Hamptons. Besides working most of your abdominal area at once, this move will help you concentrate on proper posture for all other strength-training moves.

a. Lie on your belly on a mat. Clasp your hands and raise your body so that you are balancing on your forearms and the balls of your feet. Your body should be parallel to the floor and your abs tight. Suck your abs in and don't drop your butt or curve your back.

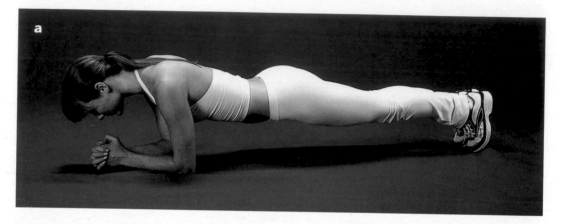

b. Inhale and raise your hips into a pike position. Lower yourself and repeat until you feel a good lower-abs burn.

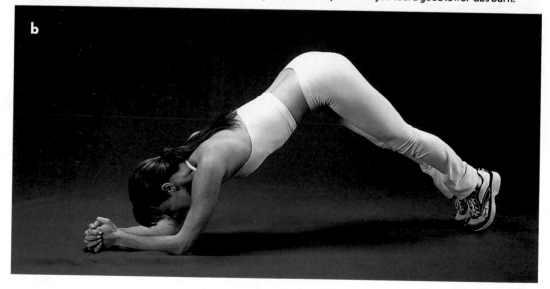

c. Finish by holding your body parallel to the floor for 30 seconds to 1 minute, then lower yourself to the starting position. If you feel this move in your lower back, you are swaying your lower back too much. Tighten your abs more.

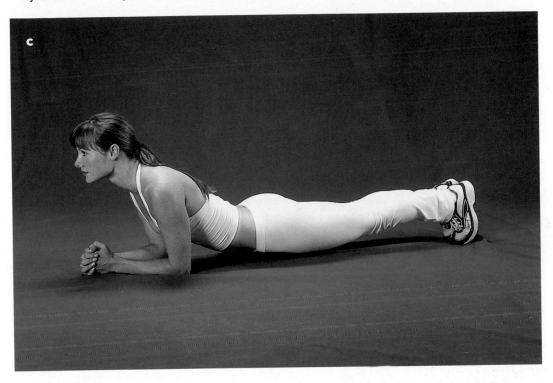

◆ Distinctively David

You can work your abs isometrically from just about any position. All you need to do is tighten them. If you're sitting in a chair, you can work them by doing a mini-crunch and tightening your abs as you do so. You can also do the same while standing. The same holds true for your obliques.

◇ ◇ ◆ ◇ ◆ ★

bicycle | internal and external obliques, rectus abdominis, lower rectus abdominis | ADVANCED

a. Lie on your back on a mat with your hands behind your head and your legs raised at a 45-degree angle from your hips. Your elbows should be out to the side far enough so that you can't see them.

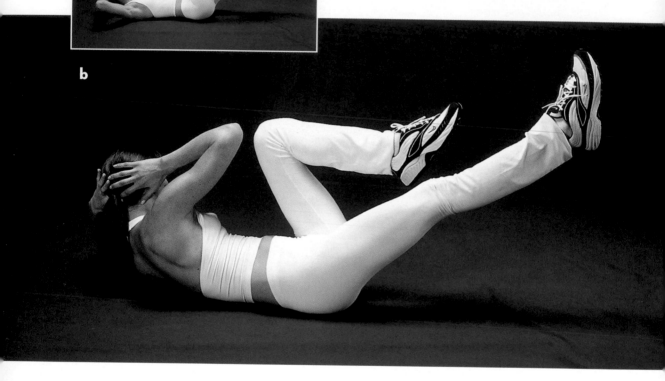

b. Exhale as you slowly bring your right elbow to your left knee. Repeat back and forth from side to side. To increase the difficulty, hold a weight behind your head.

Throughout this move, stay coordinated. Don't move your knees and elbows randomly. You're not a washing machine. If you get dizzy, you're moving your head too much.

◆Distinctively David

Depending on how you do them, bicycles can be either an effective isolated finishing burn to an abs or cardio workout, or a complete waste of time. There is no middle ground. Moving slowly is the key to doing bicycles correctly. Focus on your abs, and think sl-o-ow, sl-o-ow, sl-o-ow as you bring your elbow to your knee. Make sure your shoulders are as up as they can be throughout the move, and think "crunch," not "spin cycle in the washing machine."

CARDIO SCULPTING

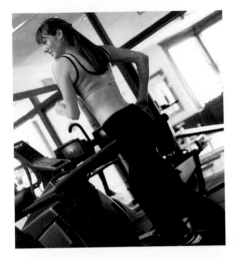

I train numerous supermodels and actresses who want to be toned and fit but *don't* want noticeable muscles. I hear this same concern from noncelebrity women who don't want to get bulky. With the right program, you can develop long, sinewy, feminine curves without looking like Gabrielle Reece or Marion Jones. (Not that they are not gorgeous, athletically beautiful specimens. They are just a little more muscular than some women want to look.)

Have I just described your exercise goals to a T? Then you'll love my cardio-sculpting exercises. These moves couple low-weight, high-repetition resistance with cardiovascular training. You'll simultaneously increase your heart and metabolic rate, burning calories and fat. You'll enhance your overall wellness, and you'll strengthen your muscles without bulk.

This routine is an amazing method of getting an efficient overall body-toning and strength workout and cardiovascular routine at the same time. It's also totally adaptable to different situations and locations.

Cardio sculpting works great for just about every body type with the exception of the stick. I recommend a 60-minute session, or 45 minutes at the very least. Do 1- to 3-minute intervals of the following series of moves interspersed with 1 to 3 minutes of treadmill running, stairstepping, jumping rope, or some other cardiovascular heart thumper. In addition to the following moves, you can also throw in some calisthenics, plyometrics, lunges, stepups, jump squats, pushups, and other moves that keep your heart rate up. Make your cardio-sculpting workout uniquely your own.

shadowboxing

A great exercise for your shoulders, back, arms, and abs, you can shadowbox with or without weights. Hold light weights in each hand, and throw a series of punches. Make sure not to punch so quickly that you hyperextend your elbows or shoulders. Throughout your workout, keep your abs tight and your shoulder blades retracted. The tighter your core, the more effective shadowboxing becomes.

Try the following punches, interspersed with some knee bends, as if you were ducking an incoming punch from your shadow.

a. Crossover. Stand with your abs tight and your back flat. Punch your left fist out diagonally, ending at torso level in front of your right ribs. Pull back and repeat on the other side.

b. Uppercut. With your left elbow against your ribs and your palm turned up, punch in an upward motion, as if you were punching someone in the stomach and trying to lift him off the ground with your fist. Pull back and repeat on the other side.

c. Hooks. Bring your bent left arm up so that it is parallel with the floor and punch with a hooking motion, as if you were trying to clock someone on the side of the jaw. Pull back and repeat on the other side.

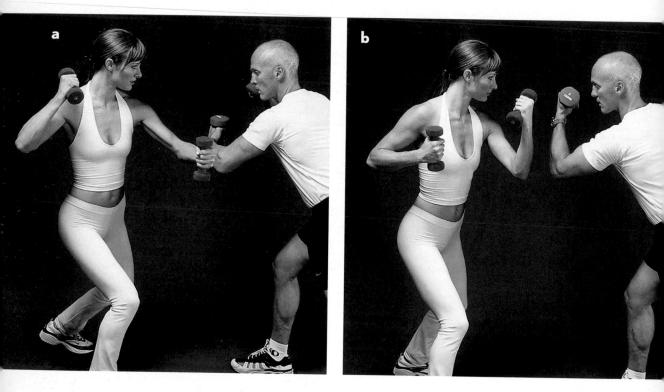

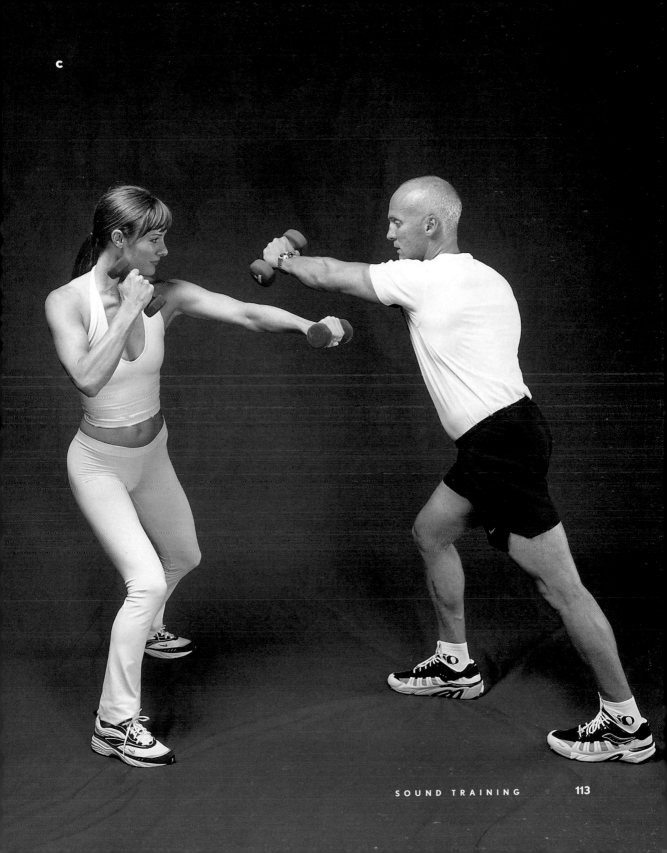

C

kicks

Add the following series of kicks to your Shadowboxing routine for a serious total-body workout. Try some Reverse Lunges (see page 66) between your Soccer Kicks and High-Knee Kicks.

a. Soccer Kick. Pretend there's a soccer ball in front of you and that you are kicking it toward the goal. Boot the ball with the inside of your right foot. Repeat with your left leg.

b. High-Knee Kick. Bring one knee in toward your chest and back to the floor. Repeat with the other leg.

c. Side Kick. Start in a squat position. As you rise, balance on your left foot and bring the knee of your right leg in toward your chest, and then kick out sideways with your right foot, with your foot flexed and heel higher than your toes. Repeat on the other side.

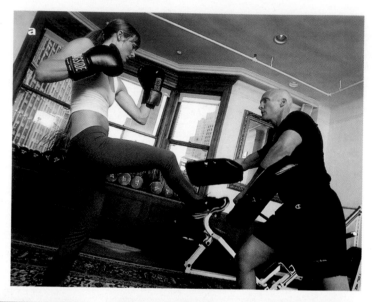

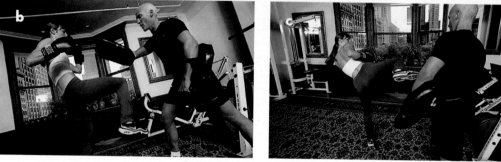

◆Try This

I call this move the Ninja Glute Blast because it looks and does exactly what the name suggests. You start by doing an asymmetrical squat with one foot placed on a step so that it's higher than the other. Once you squat down, place your body weight into the leg raised on the step and lift your other leg off the floor, bringing the knee into your chest and out to the side for a side kick. It'll get your heart pumping and your glutes burning. Once you get the move down, you can combine it with an upper-body exercise, such as a Side Lateral (see page 84).

The Right Combination

When some people train, they do multiple sets of the same exercise, resting for a minute or two between sets. I find this method of training both boring and inefficient. Rather than repeat the same exercise over and over again, I prefer to combine different exercises into one set, blasting the part of my body that I'm targeting. Not only do these combinations keep workouts interesting, they also save time because I don't have to rest between moves. I simply move fluidly from one exercise into another. And because they also target slightly different areas of my muscles, combination moves help me achieve better results.

Throughout my exercise descriptions and within the programs I've designed for you, I list many of my favorite combinations. But I challenge you to make your workout uniquely yours by designing your own signature combination moves. Here are five types of combination moves. Once you understand the theory behind each type, you'll easily be able to combine the moves in my program to consistently keep your training fresh.

Pre-exhaust. When you "pre-exhaust," you work smaller areas of a muscle before your work the muscle as a whole. For example, if you are working your chest, you would do a Dumbbell Fly, which works on shaping your chest muscles, before a Dumbbell Bench Press, which works a larger area of your chest. If you were working your biceps, you would do a Concentration Curl before a standard Biceps Curl.

Supersets and giant sets. A superset includes two moves for the same body part. A giant set includes three or more. For example, a giant set for the legs would include Squats/Knee Bends, Forward Lunges, Reverse Lunges, and sissy squats.

Drop sets. When you do a drop set, you work the same exercise first with a heavy weight and then with a lighter weight, without resting in between. For example, if you can bench press a pair of 25-pound dumbbells, you would continue to bench-press a pair of 20- or 15-pound dumbbells once you reach exhaustion.

Pyramids. The opposite of drop sets, pyramids involve working first with lighter weights and then moving to heavier weights. As the weight increases, your repetitions per set decrease.

Push-pull. Push-pull involves working opposite muscle groups such as your chest and back or your biceps and triceps. These moves are considered opposite because one is contracting, or "pushing," while the other is stretching, or "pulling."

YOUR PROGRAM

My mantra has always been, "One body, one at a time." What I mean is this: No two people have the same body or the same goals. Therefore, no two people should complete the same workout or follow the same workout schedule.

In other words, if you're a skinny guy looking to build serious muscle size and density, you're not going to follow the same weight-lifting program as a woman looking to slim down and firm up. If you're a woman with a pear-shaped body, you're not going to follow the same program as a woman with an apple-shaped body.

If you were in my club, I'd ask you a series of questions to gauge your lifestyle habits and your personal goals, and then I'd design a program unique to your needs. But I can't invite every person who buys this book into my club. So I came up with the next best thing: workout programs that address the needs of the five most common body types.

◆ **The apple.** This is your body type if you carry most of your body weight in your belly, back, and arms. Your legs are relatively thin. The apple program focuses on toning the torso area, staying away from any strength moves that could add size to the back, belly, and arms.

The apple's program involves a combination of fat-burning cardio-sculpting moves, upper-body movements, and some leg exercises for toning and shaping. I rarely suggest Basic Crunches for apples; the last thing an apple wants is a thicker midsection. Lower abdominal work and oblique work are the keys to the apple's success.

The best weight-lifting moves for the apple elongate and tone the torso area. Pullovers do this best and are an absolute essential to the apple's success. The apple's program also includes many squats, Plié Squats, cardio-boxing, front and side jumping jacks with dumbbells, Dumbbell Flies supersetted with Dumbbell Presses, Pullovers supersetted with prone Dumbbell Rows, Side Laterals, Front Raises, Upright Overhead Triceps Extensions, Skull Crushers, and Oblique and Reverse Crunches.

The best cardio moves for the apple will work the upper and lower body simultaneously. They include jumping rope, jumping jacks, power walking with dumbbells, the rowing machine, the elliptical trainer, the Versaclimber, squat thrusts, and running up stairs while holding dumbbells.

◆ **The pear.** You're a pear if you carry most of your body weight in your hips, butt, and thighs, but have a fairly flat belly. The pear's weight-lifting program focuses on combination moves that keep the heart rate up and simultaneously strengthen your lower body without adding girth. That means lots of toning—not strength—moves for the inner and outer thighs, glutes, and upper quads.

Many pears also need to tone their upper arms as well as develop their shoulders to balance out their hips. That means strength moves for the shoulders and toning for the upper arms and back.

Good weight-lifting moves for the pear include David's Deluxe Lunge Routine, Plié Squats, Wall Squats, Dead Lifts, Bench Stepups, David's Donkey Deluxe, hip floor work, combination pushups (Reverse with Standard, for example), Crunches, calisthenics, plyometrics, Dips on a Bench, Triceps Kickbacks, the Dumbbell Fly and Press combo, the Side Lateral into Front Raise combo, the Sumo Lunge with Side Lateral combo, and Pelvic Tilts.

The best cardio moves for the pear get the heart rate up without adding thigh size. They include jumping jacks, jogging in place, squat thrusts, the elliptical trainer, rowing machine, Versaclimber, jumping rope, and power walking. Avoid cycling and stairclimbing, which can both overdevelop a pear's legs, the quadriceps in particular.

◆ **The stick.** Common in men, you're a stick if despite your best efforts, you can't seem to build any noticeable muscle. Much of the stick's predicament is nutrition-related. You simply need to eat more.

In the gym, you must focus on a core strength program that focuses on your back, chest, and legs. Don't waste time working smaller muscle groups such as your arms, shoulders, and calves, especially for the first few weeks of your program. The fundamental core exercises are what you need to build that muscle.

Those moves include squats, pullups, chest presses, rows, Pullovers, Stiff-Leg Dead Lifts, and Military/Shoulder Presses.

The last thing the stick wants to do is burn more calories. So for the first few weeks, your program is only 3 days a week and contains minimal cardio. You need to warm up with cardio before lifting, so just keep the intensity low. Since cardiovascular exercise conditions your heart, it's a good idea to work in 20 minutes three times a week of low-intensity aerobic exercise.

◆ **Round.** Not to be confused with the apple, the round body type is simply a symmetrical person who is overweight or large framed. When you are heavy all over with no defining body shape, you fall into the round category.

Your program will focus on cardiovascular moves that will get your heart rate up into that fat-burning zone and tone muscle at the same time. In other words: lots of toning and cardio sculpting with low weight and high repetitions that work your entire body.

Thirty to 60 minutes of my cardio-sculpting program is your ideal workout, but you'll need to work up to that, especially if you're very overweight or very out of shape. You might start by walking around the block or at work whenever you get the chance to build your aerobic capacity. Once you can increase the intensity and duration, vary your routine as much as possible, using the treadmill, elliptical trainer, rowing machine, and Versaclimber.

The symmetrically fit person. If you've been exercising for a while and are at your goal weight but are looking for the extra edge in toning, then you fall into this body type. Overall, your body type is symmetrical, without one part calling too much attention to itself.

Your program will focus on advanced combination moves that target all of your major muscle groups equally. You need variety. All of the moves in my program are good, but switch the sequence around as much as possible. Try to train two body parts per day, working your legs twice a week. For example, one day might include chest and back exercises. The next legs and abs, and the next shoulders, arms, and legs. Work your moves into giant combination-move supersets or drop sets.

Good cardiovascular moves for fit types include the rowing machine

with the goal of going for 1,000 meters, 2,500 meters, and then 5,000 meters. Also, try the Versaclimber as well as sprints on the treadmill.

YOUR WEEK-BY-WEEK WORKOUT PLAN

Ready to get started? On the following pages, you'll find a workout program designed for each body type. Simply find your type and do the exercises indicated, according to the suggested schedule. Page numbers of the appropriate exercises are provided. (I'm sure you already remember exercises like jumping jacks and squat thrusts from elementary school gym class.)

If you are a beginner, do just one set of each exercise for Weeks 1 and 2, then do two or three sets, either by running through your routine two or three times without resting (great for apples, pears, and round types trying to lose weight) or by resting for 45 seconds to 1 minute between each set of each exercise (great for stick and fit types trying to lift heavy weights and build muscle). If you're an advanced lifter, start with three or four sets of each exercise.

During Week 1, get used to the moves and the flow of your program. I'll give you specific instructions for increasing the effectiveness of your program as the weeks progress.

Once you start to get the hang of your program, you're ready to up the ante in Week 2. You'll continue to train 5 days a week unless you're a stick, in which case you'll work out only three times a week to make sure you're not burning too many calories. If you're the round type, you'll benefit from an extra day of cardio, totaling 6 days of exercise per week. (Anyone looking for serious weight loss should work in additional cardiovascular exercise whenever possible, starting with 20 to 30 minutes three times a week and advancing to 30 to 45 minutes 3 to 6 days a week.) The other days are for rest.

By Week 3, all of the moves in my program should feel somewhat familiar. It's time to increase your resistance and your intensity. Start pushing yourself by following the specific tips I've given for each body type.

As you continue your now-regular workout, somewhere between weeks 4 and 6 you'll start seeing distinct changes in your body type. If you're a stick, you'll start filling out. If you're round, you'll be shaping up. If you're a pear or an apple, you'll re-proportion your weight. If you're fit, you'll look more toned than ever. You'll remember from chapter 2 that one of the keys to motivation is setting numerous goals. Once your body starts responding to your program, it's time for you to start addressing another goal. In "Week 4 and Beyond—The Sound Training Program" on page 130, I provide a list of popular pet peeves and a workout regimen for how to deal with each of them.

Remember: Before you start lifting on any given day, warm up with 5 to 10 minutes of cardio followed by some stretching. And, you'll get the best results if you combine the right amount of strength moves with the right amount of toning moves for your type.

The Sound Training Program—Apple

Week 1

Day 1
Standard Pushup (p. 45)
Oblique Crunch (p. 102)
Squat/Knee Bend (p. 54)
Standard Dumbbell Bench Press (p. 47)
Jumping Jack

Day 2
Reverse Crunch (p. 103)
One-Arm Dumbbell Row (p. 76)
Pullover (p. 79)
Reverse Crunch (p. 103)
Stiff-Leg Dead Lift (p. 57)
Jumping Rope

Day 3
Side Lateral (p. 84)
Front Raise (p. 85)
Military/Shoulder Press (p. 83)
Jumping Jack
Bench Stepup with Kick and Extension (p. 74)
Dips on a Bench (p. 97)
Biceps Curl (p. 90)
Oblique Crunch (p. 102)

Day 4
Squat Thrust
Advanced Incline Dumbbell Fly Press (p. 51)
Shadowboxing (p. 112)
Good Morning (p. 81)
Reverse Crunch (p. 103)

Day 5
Oblique Crunch (p. 102)
David's Deluxe Lunge Routine (p. 66)
Partial Dead Lift (p. 58)

Week 2

You can either run through your Week 1 program again, or pick new moves as substitutes, as long as they work the same body parts for that day. Focus on increasing the tempo of each workout by slowly introducing cardio sculpting and supersets into your program.

Day 1
Squat Thrust
Standard Dumbbell Bench Press (p. 47)
Dumbbell Fly (p. 50)
Jumping Jack
Oblique Twist (p. 104)
David's Deluxe Lunge Routine (p. 66)
Running in place
African Dance Step (p. 104)
Bench Stepup with Kick and Extension (p. 74)

Day 2
Scissors Reverse Crunch (p. 106)
One-Arm Dumbbell Row (p. 76)
Pullover (p. 79)
Leg Circles (p. 107)
Shadowboxing (p. 112)
Stiff-Leg Dead Lift (p. 57)
Good Morning (p. 81)

Day 3
Side Lateral (upright and bent over) (p. 84)
Torso Turn (p. 105)
Jumping Jack
Biceps Curl (p. 90)
David's Press (p. 86)
Dips on a Bench (p. 97)
David's Reverse Crab (p. 98)
Jumping Jack
Torso Turn (p. 105)

Day 4
Jumping Jack
Deluxe Pushup Routine (p. 46)
Advanced Incline Dumbbell Fly Press (p. 51)
Good Morning (p. 81)
David's Isometric Ab (p. 108)
Jump Squat
Bent-Over Dumbbell Row (p. 77)
Under-Handed Dumbbell Row (p. 78)

Shadowboxing (p. 112)
Kicks (p. 114)

Day 5
Bicycle (p. 110)
Oblique Crunch (p. 102)
Side Lunge Deluxe (p. 67)
David's Platypus Walk (p. 72)
Bench Stepup with Kick and Extension (p. 74)

Week 3

Push the tempo of your workout to keep your calorie burn high. Try to rest very little between exercises, either doing cardio moves or working opposite muscles (such as chest and back) so you don't need a rest. Also, start adding giant sets to your routine of three or more exercises in a row without a rest for the same muscle group.

Remember that Reverse Crunches are a key move for you. Intersperse them throughout your workout so that you're doing multiple sets of them by the time you finish. In addition to your weight workout, add as much cardio to your daily routine as possible by power walking with dumbbells or climbing steps with dumbbells.

Day 1
Jumping Rope
Dumbbell Fly (p. 50)
Standard Dumbbell Bench Press (p. 47)
Pullover (p. 79)
Jumping Rope
African Dance Step (p. 104)
David's Crab Crawl (p. 71)
David's Platypus Walk (p. 72)
Jumping Rope
Plié Squat with Calf Raise (p. 55)
Wall Squat with Ball (p. 56)
Jumping Rope
Oblique Crunch (p. 102)

Day 2
Reverse Crunch (p. 103)
Jumping Jack

Good Morning (p. 81)
Bent-Over Dumbbell Row (p. 77)
Under-Handed Dumbbell Row (p. 78)
Jumping Jack
Scissors Reverse Crunch (p. 106)
Superman (p. 80)
Reverse Crunch (with ball) (p. 103)

Day 3
Shadowboxing (p. 112)
Side Lateral (p. 84)
Front Raise (p. 85)
One-arm David's Press (p. 86)
Shadowboxing (p. 112)
Biceps Curl (p. 90)
Hammer Curl (p. 93)
Upright Triceps Overhead Extension (p. 96)
Dips on a Bench (p. 97)
Shadowboxing (p. 112)
David's "The Chicken" (p. 88)
Shadowboxing (p. 112)
Oblique Twist (p. 104)
African Dance Step (p. 104)

Day 4
Standard Pushup (p. 45)
Squat Thrust
Incline Dumbbell Bench Press (p. 47)
Pullover (p. 79)
Incline Dumbbell Fly (p. 52)
Squat Thrust
Reverse Crunch (p. 103)
Squat Thrust
Incline Pushup (p. 46)
One-Arm Dumbbell Row (p. 76)

Day 5
Walking Lunge (p. 66)
Oblique Twist (p. 104)
Jumping Rope
Sumo Lunge (p. 66)
African Dance Step (p. 104)
Frog Jump (p. 70)
Jumping Rope

The Sound Training Program—Pear

Week 1

Day 1
David's Deluxe Floor Routine (p. 64)
Jumping Jack
Basic Crunch (p. 101)
Reverse Crunch (p. 103)
Plié Squat with Calf Raise (p. 55)
Standard Pushup (p. 45)

Day 2
Skull Crusher (p. 94)
Close-Grip Pushup (p. 46)
Bench Stepup with Kick and Extension (p. 74)
Oblique Crunch (p. 102)

Day 3
David's Donkey Deluxe (p. 68)
Side Lunge Deluxe (p. 65)
Reverse Crunch (p. 103)
Standard Pushup (p. 45)

Day 4
Good Morning (p. 81)
Pullover (p. 79)
Upright Triceps Overhead Extension (p. 96)
Front Raise (p. 85)
Side Lateral (p. 84)

Day 5
Squat Thrust
David's Reverse Prone Scissors (p. 63)
Abs Deluxe (p. 103)
Wide Plié Squat with Calf Raise (p. 55)

Week 2

You can either run through your Week 1 program again, or pick new moves as substitutes, as long as they work the same body parts for that day. Just remember to always do toning moves for your legs, never strength moves. Increase your multiple lunge moves, combining two or three different lunges together into one set. Add some plyometric moves into your program, such as Leaping Lunges and Frog Jumps.

Day 1
David's Deluxe Lunge Routine (p. 66)
Frog Jump (p. 70)
Reverse-Grip Pushup (p. 99)
Standard Pushup (p. 45)
Double Crunch (p. 103)
David's Donkey Deluxe with Scissors (p. 68)
Standard Dumbbell Bench Press (p. 47)
Dumbbell Fly (p. 50)

Day 2
Bicycle (p. 110)
Upright Triceps Overhead Extension (p. 96)
Dips on a Bench (p. 97)
African Dance Step (p. 104)
Oblique Twist (p. 104)
Close-Grip Press
Close-Grip Pushup (p. 46)
David's Reverse Crab (p. 98)

Day 3
Plié Squat (p. 55)
David's Platypus Walk (p. 72)
Cardio Kickboxing
Reverse Crunch (with bent legs) (p. 103)
Deluxe Pushup Routine (p. 46)
Incline Dumbbell Bench Press (p. 48)
Reverse Crunch (with straight legs) (p. 103)
Side Lunge Deluxe (p. 67)

Day 4
Dips on a Bench (p. 97)
David's Reverse Crab (p. 98)
Side Lateral (p. 84)
Front Raise (p. 85)
Side Lateral (bent over) (p. 84)

Bent-Over Dumbbell Row (p. 77)
Under-Handed Dumbbell Row (p. 78)
Good Morning (p. 81)

Day 5
David's Deluxe Lunge Routine (p. 66)
Oblique Crunch (p. 102)
Prone Leg Curl (p. 62)
David's Reverse Prone Scissors (p. 63)
David's Isometric Ab (p. 108)
Jogging in place
David's Donkey Deluxe (p. 68)
Side Kick (p. 114)

Week 3

Your pear bottom should be shaping up nicely, and now you are ready for a real butt, hip, and thigh blast. For all of your leg-sculpting moves, add ankle weights if you haven't already.

Day 1
Plié Squat (p. 55)
Leaping Squat (p. 56)
Reverse Pulsing Lunge (p. 66)
Leg Circles (p. 107)
Incline Dumbbell Bench Press (p. 48)

Incline Dumbbell Fly (p. 52)
Double Crunch (p. 103)

Day 2
Skull Crusher (p. 94)
Close-Grip Press
Oblique Twist (p. 104)
David's Reverse Crab (p. 98)
Jumping Rope

Day 3
Bench Stepup with Kick and Extension (p. 74)
Reverse Lunge (p. 66)
Asymmetrical Lunge (p. 66)
David's Reverse Prone Scissors (p. 63)
Reverse Crunch (p. 103)
Decline Dumbbell Bench Press (p. 49)
Decline Dumbbell Fly (p. 52)

Day 4
Rest and eat well

Day 5
50-Yard Dash
David's Platypus Walk (p. 72)
David's Isometric Ab (p. 108)
Frog Jump (p. 70)
50-Yard Dash
Scissors Reverse Crunch (p. 106)

The Sound Training Program—Stick

Week 1

Day 1
Standard Pushup (p. 45)
Knee Bend (p. 54)
Basic Crunch (p. 101)
Standard Dumbbell Bench Press (p. 47)
One-Arm Dumbbell Row (p. 76)
Oblique Crunch (p. 102)
Reverse Crunch (p. 103)

Day 2
Eat well

Day 3
Squat (p. 54)
Reverse Crunch (p. 103)
Stiff-Leg Dead Lift (p. 57)
Incline Pushup (p. 46)
Pullover (p. 79)

Day 4
Eat well

Day 5
Military/Shoulder Press (p. 83)
Side Lateral (p. 84)
Front Raise (p. 85)
Incline Dumbbell Bench Press (p. 48)
Standard Pushup (p. 45)

Week 2

Stick to a 3-day-a-week schedule; you want to put on weight, not burn so many calories that you take it off. Keep doing the cardio moves to condition your heart, but keep the intensity low: Brisk walking is fine; running is not. Continue to focus on strength moves for your chest, back, and legs during every workout. Add more strength moves this week and increase the amount of weight you lift. Rest 45 to 60 seconds between sets, and do multiple sets of each exercise.

Try a drop set routine where you start with heavy weight and increase the reps as you decrease the weight.

Day 1
Drop set of each exercise:
Standard Pushup (p. 45)
Squat/Knee Bend (p. 54)
Basic Crunch (p. 101)
Standard Dumbbell Bench Press (p. 47)
One-Arm Dumbbell Row (p. 76)
Reverse Crunch (p. 103)

Day 2
Eat well

Day 3
Squat/Knee Bend (p. 54)
Basic Crunch (p. 101)
Stiff-Leg Dead Lift (p. 57)
Partial Dead Lift (p. 58)
Pullup
Incline Pushup (p. 46)
Pullover (p. 79)

Day 4
Eat well

Day 5
Military/Shoulder Press (p. 83)
Side Lateral (p. 84)
Front Raise (p. 85)
Incline Dumbbell Bench Press (p. 48)
Standard Pushup (p. 45)

Week 3

By now you should be putting on some size, so take your program to another level by adding multiple pyramid sets of each exercise. (Increase the weight and decrease the reps with each set.) Also, it's time for you to add workout days to your schedule.

Day 1

Standard Dumbbell Bench Press (p. 47)
One-Arm Dumbbell Row (p. 76)
Decline Dumbbell Bench Press (p. 49)
Pullover (p. 79)
Skull Crusher (p. 94)
Close-Grip Press

Day 2

Military/Shoulder Press (p. 83)
Squat/Knee Bend (p. 54)
David's Press (p. 86)
Reverse Lunge (p. 66)
Side Lateral (p. 84)
Stiff-Leg Dead Lift (p. 57)
Partial Dead Lift (p. 58)

Day 3

Power Walking
Basic Crunch (p. 101)

Day 4

Incline Dumbbell Bench Press (p. 48)
Incline Dumbbell Fly (p. 52)
Dips on a Bench (p. 97)
Triceps Kickback (p. 95)
One-Arm Dumbbell Row (p. 76)
Under-Handed Dumbbell Row (p. 78)

Day 5

Jumping Jack
Shadowboxing (p. 112)
Side Lateral (p. 84)
Sumo Lunge (p. 66)
Front Raise (p. 85)
One-Arm David's Press (p. 86)

The Sound Training Program—Round

Week 1

Day 1
Knee Bend (p. 54)
Standard Pushup (p. 45)
Jumping Jack
Basic Crunch (p. 101)
Standard Dumbbell Bench Press (p. 47)
Reverse Crunch (p. 103)
David's Deluxe Floor Routine (p. 64)

Day 2
Good Morning (p. 81)
Squat Thrust
Side Lateral (p. 84)
Front Raise (p. 85)

Day 3
Bench Stepup with Kick and Extension (p. 74)
Shadowboxing (p. 112)
Dumbbell Fly (p. 50)
Incline Dumbbell Bench Press (p. 48)
Sumo Lunge (p. 66)
Pullover (p. 79)
Upright Triceps Overhead Extension (p. 96)
Reverse Crunch (p. 103)

Day 4
David's Press (p. 86)
Side Lateral (upright and bent over) (p. 84)
Biceps Curl (p. 90)
Jumping Jack with dumbbells

Day 5
Ninja Glute Blast (p. 114)
Wide Plié Squat (p. 55)
Triceps Kickback (p. 95)
Dips on a Bench (p. 97)
Oblique Crunch (p. 102)
Reverse Crunch (p. 103)

Week 2

You can either run through your Week 1 program again, or pick new moves as substitutes, as long as they work the same body parts for that day.

Increase your cardio intensity, completing at least 20 to 30 minutes of cardio 3 or 4 days a week. Take less rest between sets, and complete more supersets and cardio-sculpting moves to keep your heart rate up throughout the workout.

Day 1
15 minutes of cardio
Side Kick (p. 114)
Side Lunge Deluxe (p. 67)
Double Crunch (p. 103)
African Dance Step (p. 104)
Bench Stepup with Kick and Extension (p. 74)
Jump Squat
Standard Pushup (p. 45)
Standard Dumbbell Bench Press (p. 47)
Dumbbell Fly (p. 50)

Day 2
Good Morning (p. 81)
Jogging in place
Jumping Jack with Side Lateral (p. 84)
Jumping Jack with Front Raise (p. 85)
Bent-Over Dumbbell Row (p. 77)
Under-Handed Dumbbell Row (p. 78)
Jogging in place

Day 3
Standard Dumbbell Bench Press (p. 47)
Close-Grip Press
Frog Jump (p. 70)
David's Platypus Walk (p. 72)
Standard Pushup (p. 45)
Close-Grip Pushup (p. 46)
Jump Squat
Jumping Rope

Day 4
Jumping Jack
Shadowboxing (p. 112)
Biceps Curl (p. 90)
Military/Shoulder Press (p. 83)
Shadowboxing (p. 112)
Concentration Curl (p. 92)
Jumping Jack with dumbbells

Day 5
Jumping Rope
Bench Stepup with Kick and Extension (p. 74)
Triceps Kickback (p. 95)
David's Deluxe Lunge Routine (p. 66)
Jumping Rope
Dips on a Bench (p. 97)
David's Reverse Crab (p. 98)
African Dance Step (p. 104)
Sumo Lunge (p. 66)
Reverse Crunch (p. 103)
Jumping Rope

Week 3

You're ready for an all-out, intense cardio-sculpting workout, complete with drop sets, pre-exhaust sets, and plyometrics. For you, every day is a sculpting day. Try to keep your heart pumping throughout your workout by resting very little between moves.

Day 1
Squat/Knee Bend (p. 54)
Side and Front Kick (p. 114)
Squat Thrust
Standard Pushup (p. 45)
Jumping Jack
Basic Crunch (p. 101)
Advanced Incline Dumbbell Fly Press (p. 51)
Reverse Crunch (p. 103)
David's Deluxe Floor Routine (p. 64)

Day 2
50-Yard Dash
Stiff-Leg Dead Lift (p. 57)
Jumping Rope
Side Lateral (p. 84)
David's Press (p. 86)
Jumping Jack

Day 3
Jumping Rope
Advanced Incline Dumbbell Fly Press (p. 51)
Incline Pushup (p. 46)
Reverse Lunge (p. 66)
Plié Squat (p. 55)
Cardio Kickboxing
Squat Thrust
Dips on a Bench (p. 97)
David's Reverse Crab (p. 98)
Jumping Rope
Standard Dumbbell Bench Press with Close-Grip
  Press (p. 47)
Jumping Rope

Day 4
Shadowboxing (p. 112)
Jumping Jack
Side Lateral (p. 84)
Front Raise (p. 85)
Shadowboxing (p. 112)
Hammer Curl (p. 93)
Biceps Curl (p. 90)
Military/Shoulder Press (p. 83)
Shadowboxing (p. 112)

Day 5
Cardio Kickboxing
Squat Thrust
Bench Stepup with Kick and Extension (p. 74)
Triceps Kickback (p. 95)
David's Donkey Deluxe (p. 68)
David's Crab Crawl (p. 71)
David's Reverse Crab (p. 98)
Leg Circles (p. 107)
Cardio Kickboxing
Oblique Twist (p. 104)

The Sound Training Program—Fit

Week 1

Day 1
Deluxe Pushup Routine (p. 46)
Reverse Crunch (p. 103)
Decline Dumbbell Press (p. 49)
Basic Crunch (p. 101)
Bench Stepup with Kick and Extension (p. 74)
Advanced Incline Dumbbell Fly Press (p. 51)
Incline Biceps Curl (p. 92)
Abs Deluxe (p. 103)

Day 2
Squat (with wide stance) (p. 54)
Crossover Lunge (p. 66)
Reverse Lunge (p. 66)
Squat Thrust
Bicycle (with ankle weights) (p. 110)

Day 3
One-Arm Dumbbell Row (p. 76)
Pullover (p. 79)
Skull Crusher (p. 94)
Dips on a Bench (p. 97)
Leg Circles (p. 107)
Double Crunch (p. 103)

Day 4
David's Press (p. 86)
Shrug (p. 87)
Side Lateral (upright and bent over) (p. 84)
Oblique Twist (p. 104)
Standard Dumbbell Bench Press (p. 47)
Dumbbell Fly (p. 50)
Incline Dumbbell Bench Press (p. 48)
Incline Dumbbell Fly (p. 52)
Deluxe Pushup Routine (p. 46)
Shadowboxing (p. 112)
Military/Shoulder Press (p. 83)

Day 5
Bench Stepup with Kick and Extension (p. 74)
Stiff-Leg Dead Lift (p. 57)
Frog Jump (p. 70)

David's Isometric Ab (p. 108)
Sumo Lunge (p. 66)
Ninja Glute Blast (p. 114)
Partial Side Lateral (p. 84)

Week 2

You can either run through your Week 1 program again, or pick new moves as substitutes, as long as they work the same body parts for that day.

For the body parts you're targeting more than once a week, make your first session a strength session (see "The Right Moves for You" on page 34 to see which exercises build strength). Then, later in the week, do a shaping/toning session (with moves from the shaping/toning column of the same chart).

This week in particular, add some push-pull combinations and drop sets (see "The Right Combination" on page 115) to your routine.

Day 1
Standard Dumbbell Bench Press (p. 47)
Pullover (p. 79)
Double Crunch (p. 103)
Incline Dumbbell Bench Press (p. 48)
Decline Dumbbell Bench Press (p. 49)
Biceps Curl (p. 90)
Reverse Crunch (with ball) (p. 103)

Day 2
Squat/Knee Bend (p. 54)
Frog Jump (p. 70)
Oblique Crunch (p. 102)
Leaping Lunge (p. 56)
Oblique Twist (p. 104)
Bench Stepup with Kick and Extension (p. 74)

Day 3
Pullup
Hanging Knee Raise
Skull Crusher (p. 94)

Basic Crunch (done on ball) (p. 101)
Triceps Kickback (p. 95)

Day 4
Jumping Jack (with light dumbbell)
Shadowboxing (with light dumbbell) (p. 112)
Incline Dumbbell Fly (p. 52)
Torso Turn (p. 105)
Decline Dumbbell Fly (p. 52)
Oblique Twist (p. 104)
Jumping Jack
Shadowboxing (p. 112)

Day 5
David's Deluxe Lunge Routine (p. 66)
Jumping Rope
David's Isometric Ab (p. 108)
Side Lunge Deluxe (p. 67)
Frog Jump (p. 70)
Plié Squat with Calf Raise (p. 55)
Jumping Rope
Double Crunch (p. 103)

Week 3

Turn your workouts upside down by adding 1 to 2 minutes of cardio moves throughout your workout. In addition, add drop sets to your routine, starting at a heavier weight and dropping to a lighter weight without rest.

Day 1
Jumping Rope
Double Crunch (p. 103)
50-Yard Dash
Deluxe Pushup Routine (p. 46)
50-Yard Dash
Standard Dumbbell Bench Press (p. 47)
Jumping Rope
Biceps Curl (p. 90)
50-Yard Dash
Double Crunch (p. 103)

Day 2
Jogging in place (with high knees)
Squat Thrust

Jogging in place (with high knees)
Jump Squat
Oblique Crunch (p. 102)
Jogging in place (with high knees)
Hanging Knee Raise
Jogging in place (with high knees)
Frog Jump (p. 70)
Leaping Lunge (p. 56)

Day 3
Rowing Machine
Pullup
Rowing Machine
Close-Grip Pushup (p. 46)
Scissors Reverse Crunch (p. 106)
Rowing Machine
Bent-Over Dumbbell Row (p. 77)
Under-Handed Dumbbell Row (p. 78)
Rowing Machine
Triceps Kickback (p. 95)
Basic Crunch (p. 101)

Day 4
Jumping Jack
Incline Dumbbell Fly (p. 52)
David's Press (p. 86)
Shadowboxing (p. 112)
Jumping Jack
Side Lateral (p. 84)
Front Raise (p. 85)
Shadowboxing (p. 112)
Torso Turn (p. 105)
Jumping Jack
African Dance Step (p. 104)

Day 5
Sumo Lunge (p. 66)
David's Deluxe Floor Routine (p. 64)
Jumping Rope
Basic Crunch (done on ball) (p. 101)
Pelvic Tilt (done on ball) (p. 73)
Jumping Rope
David's Donkey Deluxe (p. 68)
Jumping Rope
Reverse Crunch (with legs straight) (p. 103)

WEEK 4 AND BEYOND—THE SOUND TRAINING PROGRAM

After you're in the habit of following the exercise program that's right for your particular body type and you feel comfortable substituting variation exercises to keep your fitness routine fresh, then you should be ready to solve specific body problems that have always bothered you.

Everyone has a pet peeve about his or her body. For me, it's my chest and arms. I was blessed with strong legs and glutes, but my chest and arms take constant attention because they can lose size quickly. For Heidi Klum, it's her rear end and her thighs. (See her boot camp on page 228 if this is also your concern.)

For Marcy Engelman, another of my clients, it's her arms. When she came to me, she told me that she merely wanted to be able to wear capped sleeves. "I didn't even ask for sleeveless because I didn't think it was possible," she later told me. "I just had those arms that hang. Now I see definition in my arms that I haven't seen in my entire life."

Often, our pet peeves change over time, usually in relation to a big event. As summer approaches, many people want to get that flat belly or perky tush. If a formal affair is in a few weeks, many women like to tone their arms for a sleeveless dress or their back and shoulders for a backless one.

From Week 4 on, you can simultaneously work on your body type and pet peeve simply by doing your usual moves and then blasting the pet peeve area twice a week with the routines I prescribe here. Once your pet peeve starts shaping up, you may notice another area on your body that needs attention. Start blasting that area once or twice a week as well. This is an ongoing process that will keep you motivated and focused for years. Depending on your fitness level, you can work on one or two pet peeves during the same workout (such as arms and butt) as long as you have the focus, stamina, and time.

Here's a list of some common pet peeves, along with a sample workouts for each.

DROOPY BUTT

You can lift that butt by performing combination movements, especially giant sets that include numerous leg exercises in a row without a break. For example, combining Reverse with Crossover Lunges is a great butt lifter. Same with Plié Squats combined with Stiff-Leg and Partial Dead Lifts.

Here are three sample workouts to add to your routine.

WORKOUT #1
- Good Morning
- Stiff-Leg and Partial Dead Lift
- Plié Squat with Calf Raise
- Squat with Side Kick
- Pelvic Tilt

WORKOUT #2
- David's Donkey Deluxe
- Lunge set including Forward Lunge, Crossover Lunge, Side Lunge, Alexandra Lunge

WORKOUT #3
- Leaping Squat
- Leaping Lunge
- David's Crab Crawl
- David's Platypus Walk

FLABBY BELLY
Tightening up those abs will take a combination of good nutrition and lots of cardiovascular exercise as well as a stepped-up ab routine. Work your abs two or three times a week with one of the following workouts. And remember: quality, not quantity. Focus on form, not the number of reps. To up the ante, you can do many of the suggested exercises with a medicine ball squeezed between your legs.

WORKOUT #1
- Crunches (all kinds)
- Oblique Twist
- Reverse Crunch (with ball)
- Leg Circles
- Bicycle (with ankle weights)

WORKOUT #2
- Leg Lift
- Oblique leg lift (with legs at a right angle)
- Oblique Crunch

WORKOUT #3
- Double Crunch
- Superman
- David's Isometric Ab

CHICKEN LEGS
Nothing cures chicken legs like squats. Do them with a regular stance (with your feet hip-width apart), a wide stance, and a narrow stance. Try the following workouts.

WORKOUT #1
- Squat (wide and narrow stances)
- Lunge (all kinds)
- Stiff-Leg and Partial Dead Lift

WORKOUT #2
- Leg Extension
- Decline Leg Curl
- Walking Lunge

WORKOUT #3
- Leg Extension
- Leg Curl
- Wide Squat
- Leaping Squat

LOVE HANDLES
The key to tightening the flab along the sides of your belly is isometric movements performed nice and slow. "Isometric" is just a fancy word that means you're contracting your muscle. Every time you suck in your abs, you're doing an isometric contraction.

Intersperse abdominal work throughout your workouts, warming up with some ab moves, breaking in the middle for some ab moves, and finishing with some ab moves. You'll need to do a lot of twisting movements to fully address your love handles, but don't get carried away by using excessive weight. That will make them thick, giving you a blocky appearance. Try the following workouts.

WORKOUT #1
◆ Oblique Twist
◆ Bicycle
◆ Leg Circles

WORKOUT #2
◆ Oblique Twist (with dumbbells)
◆ Torso Turn with Twist
◆ African Dance Step

WORKOUT #3
◆ Hanging Knee Raise with Twist
◆ Vertical Bicycle (with ankle weights)
◆ David's Isometric Ab
◆ Oblique Crunch

FLABBY ARMS
To firm up your arms, you must attack your biceps and triceps from all directions. That's why I suggest doing so many different types of curls and presses. They all work slightly different parts of your arm muscles.

WORKOUT #1
◆ Close-Grip Pushup
◆ Skull Crusher
◆ Close-Grip Press

WORKOUT #2
◆ Deluxe Pushup Routine
◆ Dips on a Bench
◆ Reverse Pushup
◆ Triceps Kickback
◆ Hammer Curl with Concentration Curl

WORKOUT #3
◆ Shadowboxing
◆ Jumping jacks (with dumbbells)
◆ David's Crab Crawl

FLABBY THIGHS
Doing at least 100 reps of combination moves such as my Donkey Deluxe will blast your thighs. You want to do lots of reps with low resistance, but you don't want the moves to be so easy that you're daydreaming. As soon as your leg movements become easy, strap on a pair of ankle weights. Try the following workouts.

WORKOUT #1
◆ David's Donkey Deluxe
◆ David's Deluxe Floor Routine
◆ Plié Squat with Calf Raise
◆ Leg Extension
◆ Leg Curl

WORKOUT #2
◆ Kicks
◆ Squat with Side Kick
◆ Stiff-Leg and Partial Dead Lifts

WORKOUT #3
◆ David's Deluxe Lunge Routine
◆ David's Crab Crawl

◆ David's Platypus Walk
◆ Frog Jumps

SCRAWNY CHEST AND ARMS

Aside from building up your strength with pushups, bench presses are also the way to go, especially if you vary the angle of the bench. Focus on lifting a heavy weight with few reps to really put on the muscle. But never lift a weight so heavy that you have to sacrifice form in the process. Try the following workouts.

WORKOUT #1
◆ Pushup (Standard and Incline)
◆ Standard Dumbbell Bench Press
◆ Incline Dumbbell Bench Press

WORKOUT #2
◆ Incline Pushup
◆ Decline Dumbbell Bench Press
◆ Incline Dumbbell Bench Press

WORKOUT #3
◆ Dips (done between two chairs)
◆ Weighted Pushup
◆ Bench Press with Dumbbell Fly (all kinds)

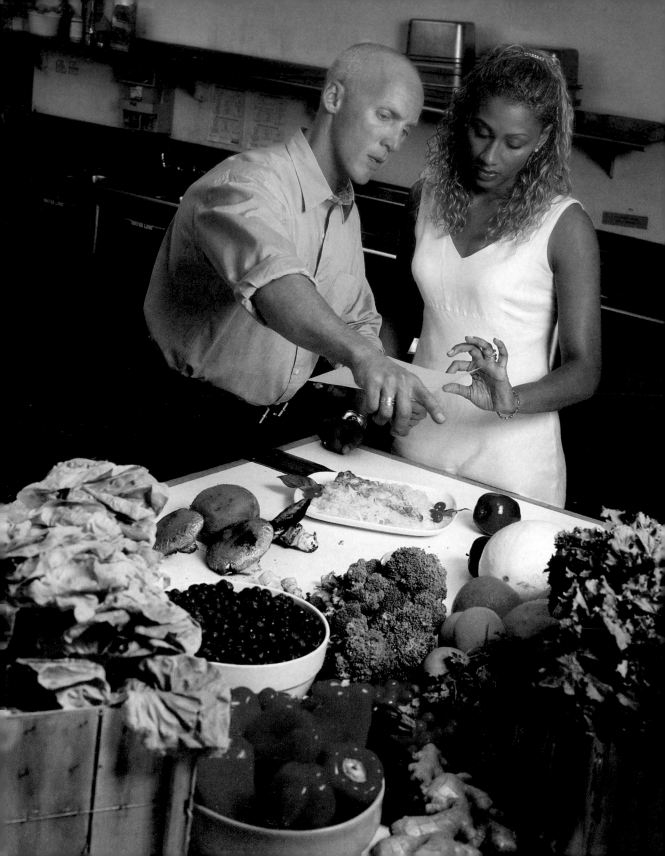

Chapter Four

SOUND EATING

IN PUBLICATIONS such as the *New York Times* and *Time* magazine, I have been called everything from the fitness and nutrition guru to the Diet Enforcer. I earned the title after clients began inviting me to dine out with them and help them make sound food choices. I've even accompanied actress and supermodel James King on modeling trips to Paris to train with her and help her eat soundly. Today, whether she's in Paris, London, or Los Angeles, she makes sound food choices, even though I'm not there.

The key word here is "choice." We all have choices. As my parents said when I was growing up, "Make the best choices out of those presented to you."

You see, it doesn't matter where you are. Whether you're eating in your own kitchen, at a restaurant, at a company cafeteria, or at a picnic, you can make better, nutritionally sound choices. Peanuts or pretzels? Tuna on whole wheat or pasta primavera? It's all about making the best choice with the options you have.

If you're a veteran calorie and fat-gram counter, my Sound Eating plan is going to make you take a leap of faith. I don't count calories. I don't count fat grams. I don't count carbs. I won't tell you to add up everything you eat into neat and tidy percentages. But I will tell you how to eat well. My eating plan will make you healthy. It will help you lose weight and feel more energized. It will help you control your eating, rather than allowing your eating to control you. It will help you eat to live, rather than live to eat. Yes, you'll pay attention to the quantity of foods you eat, but you'll also pay attention to the quality of those foods.

My Sound Mind, Sound Body program will help clear your mind and body of clutter so that you can more easily listen to your body's voice. It will tell you when you need sustenance.

It has worked for me. It's worked for my family. It's worked for my clients. Now it will work for you.

WHY WE EAT THE WAY WE DO

Before you roll your eyes and think that I was raised in a monastery where I ate only the sparest portions of food, sit back and I'll tell you a little story.

I was raised in a traditional Jewish suburban household. The kitchen was everything to us. When we ate, we were never allowed to watch television. The focus was on the food and on each other. Discussions, family meetings, crisis interventions, and party planning all took place around the kitchen table, accompanied by the requisite coffee (enough to alter the coffee futures market at times), tea or milk and cookies, cakes, or Danishes, all made by my food-obsessed grandmother who constantly made us feel that we should be in-

credibly grateful for every morsel of food we had.

My grandmother grew up in Latvia where she was orphaned as a young child. She was forced to move from the care of one family member to another. Money and food were scarce. Nobody carved every last bit of meat off the bone like my grandmother did. She ate parts that my sisters and I thought inedible.

My grandmother helped raise us kids since my mother, like many moms in the 1960s and 1970s, worked. For every meal, my grandmother served three or four courses. Dinners always started with an appetizer—fruit, stuffed cabbage, matzoh ball soup—followed by an entrée of either meat or poultry, vegetables, and a starch. If you were still able to sit upright after that, there was dessert. "You do not have to be hungry for dessert," as Grandma often said.

If we just couldn't stuff that last morsel in our mouths, Grandma would tell us stories about starving children. My sisters and I were tempted to find a way to transport unwanted food to those children. Surely they could use some of Grandma's cake or cooked fruit.

After 17 years of eating like this, it was quite a shock to my system when I went off to college. In that first semester, as other students were gaining the freshmen 15, I *lost* 15 pounds. While other students were busy learning about beer bongs, I was finally discovering my body's voice and clock. It was during my freshman year that I realized that the path to my Sound Mind and Sound Body had been cluttered with poor nutrition. It didn't take long for me to realize that the pains in my stomach I often had while growing up was my body saying, "What's up with all this food?"

Now, even as I lost this weight, I was not starving myself. In fact, my mother, who lived nearby, delivered my groceries by placing them through my ground-floor bedroom dorm window. This led to many interesting moments, especially one particular morning when my girlfriend awakened me because a well-manicured hand was reaching through the window.

While at college, I learned to eat when I was hungry and stop when I was full. Sure, I had binges. There's nothing like cold pizza at 3:00 A.M. or cookies and milk before bed. But I was beginning to discover that food, if approached healthfully, could make me feel stronger and more alert, and also help me grow much-needed muscles.

Now, 23 years later, I have reached a point in my life where I can say that I fully understand the relationship of the mind and body, and how food can easily alter the delicate balance between the two. Feeding the mind-body machine with the proper foods, nutrients, vitamins, and supplements is an integral part of the process.

Like me, you may overeat because of "family training." Or maybe you overeat because of stress, boredom, loneliness, exhaustion, or some other emotion or circumstance. Your first step toward more Sound Eating will be a matter of recognizing the reasons you overeat and addressing them.

TAKING CONTROL

A baby cries and a mother doesn't know what to do, so she sticks a bottle in the baby's mouth. You come home from school with a good report card and are rewarded with your favorite meal. You've just been dumped by your significant other—yeah, yeah, yeah, you get the drill—you head for the vanilla swiss almond ice cream.

We are conditioned at an early age to believe that food will be the answer—our sustenance, our comfort, our celebration. Do you often think about food? Do you count every calorie that you eat? Do you eat to soothe your feelings? Do you go to the freezer for a ½ cup of ice cream only to eat the whole pint? Then, like many people, you are also a disorderly eater.

You can, however, gain control over food. You can eat to give yourself energy in the afternoon rather than eat to numb the stress of the morning. As one of my clients put it: "I'm more cognizant of taking care of my body as a whole and realizing that it needs good fuel. Before I was trying not to eat fast food because I knew it was fattening. Now I'm eating good food because I know it's good fuel and good for me in general. I try to eat foods that will give me energy and support my program, food that will help me function on a higher level."

One of the first steps to gaining that control is admitting that you're not a perfect eater—and never will be. Life is too short to be totally deprived. The key to Sound Eating is

Step Up to Sound Eating

Step 1. Change your eating environment to encourage yourself to pay attention to how and what you eat. Always eat while sitting down with your food on a plate in front of you on a table. Never eat while watching television or reading the paper, and until you gain more control, try to eat alone, not with other people. The goal is to truly enjoy your food.

Step 2. Once you've changed your environment, you're ready to change what's on your plate. Could you get the same satisfaction out of something that's a little healthier? For example, if you are craving pizza, blot off the oil, or ask for light cheese or no cheese. Take off some of the cheese. Don't eat the crust. Or make your own with veggie pepperoni and veggie cheese. Each of those choices will create a more healthy meal.

Step 3. Now add joy to eating. Try to chew your food as long as possible before swallowing. Smell it. Look at it. Taste it. Treat everything you eat as if it were the best that money can buy.

Step 4. Once you've learned to savor your food, start paying attention to your body as you eat. Are you actually hungry when you start eating? When does that hunger go away? Try to stop eating once you've satisfied your hunger. Try to always leave some food on your plate. Never leave the table feeling stuffed. By eating slowly, you allow your belly to send the "I'm full" message to your brain most efficiently. Otherwise, there is a delay, and once your belly starts aching from overeating, it's already too late.

Step 5. Pay attention to the times when you eat and the times when you are not hungry. Why are you eating? What drove you to those chips, cookies, or doughnuts? Was it anger, stress, depression, frustration? Figure out the cause and take steps to address it proactively.

balance and moderation. Striving to eat better than you did yesterday is always a good goal. But striving to never ever eat pasta, bagels, candy, or fatty steak will set you up for bingeing and disappointment.

One night while working on this book, I started craving pizza. The craving began when I was writing about pizza. I didn't give in because I thought it would go away. But as each day passed and I still wanted some pizza, I knew I had to have some.

So one night, I stayed in to write, and I ordered a pizza and a salad. For whatever reason, the pizza just didn't measure up to my fantasy, so I stopped eating it after one slice. Why go on eating such a fatty and carb-laden food when I'm not enjoying it?

That's the key to making your food choices: enjoyment. Presence of mind and body. Attention to taste, texture, and satisfaction. Go ahead and have some pizza, cheesecake, chocolate, or whatever else you are craving. But savor it. Taste it. Chew it. Smell it. Remember: one or two cookies are okay. Half a box is not.

Many of my clients are unconscious eaters, particularly when they get nervous. They don't even notice that they are putting food in their mouths. They can eat a dozen doughnuts or 2 pints of ice cream in one sitting.

If you can't resist snacking at night, begin substituting healthier foods. For example, instead of ice cream, have wheat germ with soy milk. It's not the perfect choice, but maybe in a few more months you'll replace your late-night snack with a small amount of peanut butter or other protein. Or maybe you'll be so under control that you won't need to eat in the "red zone" (see "What to Eat, and When" on page 158) at all.

CHOOSING FOODS

Once you're in control of your eating, you're ready to make Sounder food choices. The Soundest choice is not necessarily the lowest-calorie choice or the lowest-fat choice. It's the choice that will fuel your body best, giving you the energy you need to complete your daily Sound Training workout as well as tackle the rest of your day with vigor.

Throughout the 1970s and 1980s—when fat was vilified—people turned to pasta, rice, bagels, and nonfat snacks when they wanted to lose weight. And most of them got fatter. While everyone was focusing on fat, they forgot about balance. They began eating foods packed with nutrient-sparse starches and sugars. The caloric wallop of many of these starchy, sugary foods was the same as their fat-laden cousins, yet people ate more of them. They ended up with a carbohydrate hangover, carb face (see "About-Face" on page 140), and feelings of lethargy and hunger.

Pasta, the "healthy" alternative to meat dishes in the 1970s and 1980s, has caused its fair share of bloated guts, saggy butts, and triglyceride readings that resemble those of a $10 million baseball player's batting average. That's because pasta is made from processed wheat. Wheat in and of itself is not bad. But once you slice off the hull and siphon off everything that makes it "whole," you're left with white flour, which has no more nutritional relevance than white sugar.

I'm not saying that you can never have pasta again. I am saying that you should think about your food choices and what effect they will have on your body.

I once went out to eat with several friends at an Italian restaurant. They all ordered pastas: gnocchi, risotto, spaghetti. I went for a salad and grilled meat. Sure, the pasta sounded appealing, but at the end of the meal, I was the only one not complaining of a bloated stomach. The next day, I was the only one

About-Face

After 6 weeks on my Sound Mind, Sound Body program, many of my clients rave about their transformed bodies. But they also notice another interesting change. Their skin looks radiant. As one of my clients put it: "When people see me, they tell me that I have a glow—a healthy, positive energy."

I like to call it the Sound Face. There are many other "faces" out there. Two notable ones are "carb face" and "zero-carb face."

Carb face. I can tell when one of my clients has recently experienced a carb binge. She'll come in looking puffy. It strikes first in the eyes, and sometimes, if the binge was bad enough, it affects the cheeks, too.

In people who are certified out-of-control carboholics, you can also see it in their abdomen. No matter how many crunches they do, no matter how skinny they starve themselves, their abs and sometimes their triceps, look flabby.

Zero-carb face. When people spend too much time eating horrible protein sources and no fruits and vegetables, they start to look sick. Their skin becomes sallow and they develop dark circles under their eyes.

So if you ever want to know if your diet is balanced, just look in the mirror. It won't lie.

without the common post-pasta malady of carb face. If you play, you pay. Knowing the consequences of your choices before you make them can often help steer you in a Sounder direction.

Remember: This isn't about deprivation. But you should strive for balance. In every meal, you should have some protein, some carbohydrate, and even a little fat. And within those three balanced food groups, you can make Sound choices.

You'll find a recurring theme as you read about Sound carbohydrate, protein, and fat choices. The Soundest food in any of those categories is the one grown or raised organically and served to you as fresh and whole as possible. The more your food resembles its natural state, the more nutrients it holds. In other words, an apple is better than applesauce, fresh spinach better than canned, a potato is better than a potato chip, and a roasted turkey breast is better than lunchmeat from a deli. Similarly, produce grown locally will give you more nutritional bang than produce grown halfway around the world. The fresher, the better.

While on vacation in Italy for a month, I ate whole foods as fresh as you can get. Each day, I picked my own produce. I went down to the docks and bought freshly caught fish. And I ate enormous meals, sometimes four of them a day.

During that month, I exercised about the same as usual, or even a little less. Yet my body fat decreased, and so did the body fat of the clients who were with me. That's the power of fresh foods. They're better for your health. They're better for your energy levels. And they're better for your waistline. Buying and eating fresh and whole foods should be the number one influence on every food choice you make.

SOUND CARBOHYDRATE CHOICES

Not long ago, my dad had a bad scare. After a routine blood test, his doctor gave him a call. My dad's triglycerides, a nasty type of fat that raises the risk for heart disease, were through the roof. His blood pressure had jumped, too. He was exhibiting all the signs of a common family trait: diabetes.

I remember calling Dad the day after he got those results. He was depressed. He couldn't understand how, after a lifetime of exercising, running, and eating relatively well, he could have such poor bloodwork results. When we analyzed his eating habits, we realized that he had been eating too many carbohydrates, especially the bad types that tend to dramatically raise blood sugar levels.

I convinced him that by cutting out, bread, cookies, potatoes, and pasta, and by eating more frequent yet smaller meals, he would see and feel immediate improvement. He replaced his cookies with protein shakes and low-carbohydrate protein bars. This helped him stabilize his blood sugar.

A month later, his blood pressure had dropped 30 points and his triglycerides had dropped by 100 points. He also lost 10 pounds.

I tell you that story not to scare you into omitting all carbohydrates, but to show you how a simple nutritional switch can go a long way toward promoting a Sound Body.

Please don't confuse my Sound Eating plan with any of a number of popular low-carbohydrate diets. They tell you that all carbohydrates are bad—even those that come from fruits and vegetables. That's simply not true. Yet it's also not true that eating all of the low-fat or nonfat carbohydrate foods you want will help you maintain a reasonable weight and good health. Rather, you must balance good carbohydrates with good proteins and fats, and not choose too much of either. If *some is good, more is not necessarily better.*

You see, all carbohydrates are not created equal. Some—found in most fruits, vegetables, and whole grains—contribute to good health and a good figure. Others—found in foods made from white sugar and white flour—tend to make you hungry, plump out your fat cells, and clog your arteries. How do you know the difference? Follow these pointers.

Get the whole picture. As I mentioned earlier, the closer your food resembles its natural state, the better its nutritional punch. Foods made from whole grains are good, but be careful. Because the Food and Drug Administration allows deceptive food labeling, some foods appear more wholesome than they really are. For example, if a package says "wheat bread," it's made mostly of white flour. A package that says "100-percent whole wheat bread" contains some white flour and some wheat flour. The best type of bread you can buy can be found in gourmet bakeries and health food stores. You'll know if your bread is truly whole grain if it's dense and heavy. If it tastes light and airy, it's made from mostly white flour.

Stay away from fake food. If the ingredient label contains a list of words you can't pronounce or define, don't eat it. If you don't know where it came from, it's probably not good for you. This is especially true with sugar substitutes such as sorbitol, saccharin, and Nutrasweet. Though I don't encourage eating lots of white sugar, if you need something sweet, sugar is better than an artifical sweetener. Raw sugar is better than white sugar.

Follow the glycemic index. The glycemic index (GI) ranks foods on a scale of 0 to 100 based on the extent to which they raise blood sugar levels immediately after eating. Foods that rank high on the index are rapidly digested and absorbed. They tend to inflict roller-coaster levels of blood sugar on your system, first giving you a rush of energy and then a crash. To maintain long-lasting energy, reduce cravings and hunger, and prevent heart disease and diabetes, you want steady blood sugar. Thus, you must primarily eat foods that rank low on the glycemic index. All proteins and fats are low glycemic foods, so you don't need to worry about meats and oils. But carbohydrates vary widely.

Generally, breakfast cereals made from wheat bran, barley, and oats are low on the GI scale. The same is true for whole grain breads that contain whole seeds. Most fruits and vegetables are low GI, with some exceptions, such as baked potatoes, parsnips, and carrots. To see where various foods rank on the GI scale, see "Know the Index" on page 145.

Watch out for hidden calories. Many people munch on carrots and grapes as if they were calorie-free. These foods, as well as a few others, have erroneously earned reputations as "diet foods." For example, one ba-nana contains 29 grams of carbohydrate and 116 calories. A ½ cup of corn gives you 20 grams of carbs and 80 calories. Just one medium baby carrot offers 8 carbohydrate grams and 32 calories. That may not seem like a lot until you consider how many baby carrots most people snack on. It's more like 10 to 15. Last, 1½ cups of grapes will set you back 24 grams and 96 calories. Again, it's not that these foods are in the same category as pasta or as butter, but they're certainly not "diet" foods.

If you don't think you can live without your starchy and processed carbs, think again. Many of my clients were carbohydrate addicts before they met me. They lived on bread, pasta, white rice, sugar, and desserts. Eve Stuart was one of them. "I had this tremendous sweet tooth," she told me 1 month after she joined my club. "That has changed. I was out to dinner last night and I looked at the dessert list. I decided to order dessert. I took a couple of bites and thought, 'I don't really like this that much anymore.' In some ways it was depressing, and in other ways it was good because it was easy not to finish it."

When you are starting from such an addicted place, it's hard to cut all starchy, processed, high-glycemic carbs on the same day. Here are some steps to take:

◆ Start by always eating some protein along with any high-glycemic, processed, or starchy carbohydrate. For example, if you're going to have a cracker, top it with some tuna. That small amount of protein will help prevent the carbohydrate binge.

◆ Make Sounder carbohydrate choices when you can. For example, switch from white bread to sourdough and then to whole grain. Also, when sweetening your food, switch from white sugar to fruit sugar (fructose), which doesn't tend to promote such a roller-coaster blood sugar response. (You can find fructose at health food stores). Also better than white sugar are raw sugar, brown sugar, honey, molasses, and maple syrup, which all contain trace minerals and tend to be binge-proof.

◆ Begin to cut back on desserts and other nutritionally vacant carbs. You can eat them in moderation. For example, a few bites of apple pie is okay. A few slices of apple pie is not. And a few slices of plain apple, without the pie, is even better.

◆ Stay away from particular types of carbohydrate foods that make you lose control.

◆ Avoid certain fruits that are particularly high in sugar and/or have a high glycemic index such as bananas, mangos, pineapple, grapes, and cherries. Yes, bananas are high in potassium, but so is cantaloupe for less sugar and calories. As I like to say, *I've never seen a skinny gorilla.*

SOUND PROTEIN CHOICES

Eating protein is the key to building lean muscle mass and lowering your hunger and cravings. That said, all forms of protein are not Sound. Some diet experts would have you believe that you can eat any form of protein and lose weight. People on these diets have gobbled down steaks, bacon, hamburgers, and spare ribs, all in the name of weight loss.

My late aunt was a great believer in eating all of the protein on her plate regardless of the quality. I mourn her loss deeply and am angered by such illogical reasoning.

High-protein diets have been criticized by many respected nutrition experts. True, most people lose weight on these diets. But they don't lose it in a healthy way. The protein and fat overload can clog your arteries, put you at risk for kidney stones, give you bad breath, and lower your immunity. It also tends to make you feel lethargic. Your muscles burn carbohydrate for fuel. Without a balanced diet that includes Sound protein, Sound carbohydrates, and Sound fats, you'll run out of energy during your workouts.

From a vanity standpoint, such a protein overload tends to cause an interesting phenomenon I call zero-carb face (see "About-Face" on page 140).

I promote Sound protein choices.

Know the Index

Here is the glycemic index of 53 common foods. Anything above 70 is in the danger zone.

Breads

Dark rye	76
White bread	70
Sourdough	57
Whole wheat bread	53
Pumpernickel	41
Heavy mixed grain	30

Cereals

Cornflakes	84
Cheerios	83
Rice Krispies	82
Puffed Wheat	80
All Bran	42

Grains

Rice, white	87
Rice, brown	76
Cream of Wheat, instant	74
Risotto	69
Oatmeal, quick	65
Basmati	58
Oatmeal, old-fashioned	49
Bulgur	48
Whole wheat spaghetti	37
Barley	25

Snack Foods

Rice cakes	82
Jelly beans	80
Mars Bar	65
Popcorn	55
Potato chips	54
Chocolate	49

Legumes

Peas	49
Baked beans	48
Chickpeas	42
Lentils	28
Soybeans	18
Peanuts	14

Vegetables

Parsnips	97
Baked potato	85
Mashed potatoes	73
Carrots	71
Beets	64
Sweet corn	55
Sweet potatoes	54

Fruits

Watermelon	72
Pineapple	66
Raisins	64
Fruit cocktail, canned	55
Banana	55
Kiwi	52
Orange	44
Grapes	43
Peach	42
Apple juice	41
Apple	38
Grapefruit	25
Plum	24

Stay away from the prime rib, London broil, and bacon. Here are some tips to guide your choices.

Go lean. Most types of protein contain some fat, and the type of fat they contain is the saturated type that tends to clog arteries. So opt for lean protein choices.

Your leanest types of meat contain the word "loin." For example, a sirloin steak is the leanest type of steak you can eat. Ground sirloin is better than ground chuck. Whatever you do, if it's an organ meat, just stay away.

When buying any type of meat, ignore the packaging that claims it's "97 percent fat-free." Meat is labeled according to fat weight, not fat calories. Fat weighs much less than muscle, as you remember from chapter 2. So a hunk of meat that's only 3 percent fat by weight might be as much as 40 or 50 percent fat as a percentage of calories.

Look at the marbling. If you can see specks of fat all through the meat, it's a fatty cut.

In poultry, the leanest meat is in the breast. When buying ground chicken or turkey, make sure to ask for 100 percent breast meat. Otherwise, you'll end up with other, fattier poultry parts.

Go wild. I encourage people to eat wild game. When animals move around and forage for their own food, they are healthier, more muscular, and less fatty. Buffalo, elk, and antelope are, on the whole, much better for you than beef.

Go for eggs. I once bought into the no-yolk craze, but research shows that yolks probably aren't as bad for you as once thought. Still, the yolk is where the egg's fat and cholesterol is stored. You can cut your calorie wallop in half by sticking with egg whites. For taste and texture, I like to mix one yolk in with a bunch of whites for omelettes and scrambled eggs.

So what do you do with extra egg yolks when you're using only whites? Freeze them. Or, if you have a relatively young dog, you can garner major points by putting one egg yolk in his food bowl.

Buy clean protein. I once had a friend who remarked, "Why do you think they call it fowl? It's because they are foul." I'm not saying you should never eat chicken or turkey— they are among your leanest protein sources. But they *are* fairly dirty birds. If you do eat poultry, go organic and free-range.

Buy organic. The agriculture industry routinely gives cattle, pigs, and poultry hormone shots to encourage faster growth and more abundant milk production. Because these unnaturally high levels of hormones tend to lower the animals' immunity, they follow up with routine antibiotic shots as well. My sister only gives her kids organic milk. You should do the same.

Buy fresh. Your best protein sources are as whole and as fresh as possible. In other words, fresh tuna from the fish store is better than tuna from the can. Fresh salmon is better than smoked. Fresh turkey breast is better than lunchmeat. In general, if it comes in a can or shrink wrap, sodium and other preservatives have been added. If you have no choice but to use canned, make sure to rinse it very well before eating.

Eat pure protein. I'm going to risk sounding crunchy-granola here, but I strongly believe that each piece of meat possesses the karmic energy from its host. If a chicken or cow or pig lived in hellish conditions before it was killed, I personally don't want to put that negative energy into my body. I grew up in a Jewish household where we ate kosher meats. Meat is kosher only if the animal it came from was, among other things, raised and butchered in the most humane way possible.

Know your fish. Fish has earned a reputation as a health food, and for the most part, that's true. Yet some types of fish are worth staying away from. For example, large carnivorous fish such as swordfish and shark tend

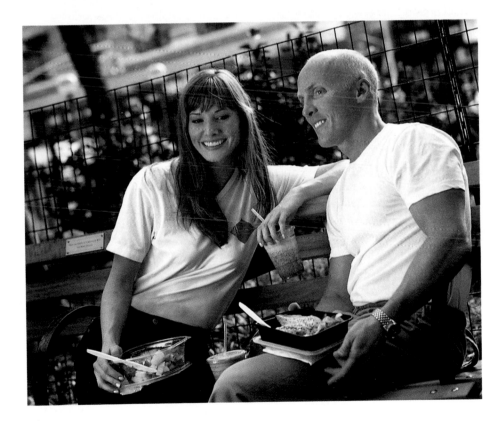

to contain high amounts of mercury and ocean pollutants. Shellfish, by nature of their eating style, also tend to take on the characteristics of the water where they live. If they live in a polluted area—and many of them do—they'll contain stuff you don't want to eat.

Beyond pollutants, some types of fish are going extinct. You can ensure you buy healthy, sustainably harvested fish by shopping online at www.ecofish.com and www.pelican-packers.com. You can also get a sustainable fish report from Environmental Defense (www.environmentaldefense.org). In general, the worst types of fish to buy include: Atlantic cod, Atlantic halibut, farmed salmon (farming pollutes and destroys wild salmon habitat), grouper, monkfish, orange roughy, Pacific rockfish, shark, prawns, skate, snapper, and swordfish.

The best for your health and your environmental sensitivity are cold-water fish that contain a special type of fat called omega-3 fatty acid. Omega-3 fats have been shown to fight heart disease, cancer, and a host of other health conditions. They may even aid in weight loss. Many of these fish swim abundantly: anchovies, Atlantic herring, bluefish, Spanish and Atlantic mackerel, sardines, striped bass, and wild Alaskan salmon. Though not high in omega-3's, catfish, mahi-mahi, Pacific halibut, and tilapia are also good environmental choices.

Cut back on dairy. Yes, milk contains lots of calcium. But it also contains a sugar called lactose that many people can't digest. Its protein, called casein, also causes coldlike symptoms in certain casein-sensitive people.

You can consume calcium from many other sources, including tofu, spinach, anchovies and sardines, almonds, broccoli, kale, mustard greens, collards, legumes, and leafy greens. If you're truly worried about getting enough calcium, you can take a supplement or consume dairy in the form of natural, organic yogurt, which contains a special type of bacteria that promotes intestinal health and aids lactose digestion.

FATS

Back in the 1980s, many people tried to eliminate fat from their diets. But scientists now have learned that fat has some important functions. It's good for your sex drive as well as your mood, among other things. It also tends to keep hunger under control.

The key to eating fat without getting fat is eating the right kinds.

Generally, all fats that come from animals—known as saturated fats—and fats that come from processed foods—known as trans fats—are bad for your health and your waistline.

These include lard, butter, margarine, beef fat, chicken fat, and milk fat as well as the hydrogenated fat in fried foods and processed foods such as doughnuts, potato chips, crackers, breakfast cereals, and just about everything that comes in a box. If you must decide whether to use butter or margarine, go for the butter. At least it comes from milk, whereas margarine is completely processed. Remember: When in doubt, go natural.

On the other hand, monounsaturated and polyunsaturated fats are good for you. Found in nuts, fatty vegetables such as avocados, fatty fish, olives and olive oil (in small amounts), flaxseeds and flaxseed products, soybeans and soy products, and other types of vegetable oils (except for palm and coconut oil). These fats have been shown to reduce heart disease, cancer, and arthritis. Eaten in the right amounts, they also may fend off depression and mood swings. And to me, they seem to dampen the appetite.

FLUIDS

Water is so important that I consider it the "lost nutrient." Many of us consistently walk around dehydrated, which leads to fatigue and headaches. When you're training, dehydration can hinder your muscle growth, in ef-

fect slowing your metabolism. You also need water to flush out all the toxins you take in during the day from polluted air to impure food.

As with protein, fat, and carbohydrate, not all fluids are created equal. Here are some tips to maximize your fluid intake.

Make water the mainstay. It has no calories. On the other hand, the average soda or fruit juice blend will set you back 100 to 200 calories as well as send your blood sugar soaring.

Drink pure water. Unless you have a filtering system, use your tap water only for showering, laundering, and dishwashing. Your drinking and cooking water should come from a bottle. My favorite brand is Fiji Natural Artesian, which is bottled 1,500 miles from the nearest continent. It has a very low mineral content (or dirt content as I like to say), giving it a nice, clean taste. Fiji Water has 160 parts per million (ppm) of dissolved solids, whereas Evian has close to three times that amount.

Avoid fluid drainers. Any beverage that contains alcohol or caffeine will discourage your intestine from absorbing water, causing you to urinate more out than you should. Keep both types of beverages to a minimum of two or fewer servings a day.

Drink Sounder wake-up beverages. I have a love/hate relationship with coffee. I love the taste. I love the smell. And I love how it makes me feel. But I don't love the stained teeth, bad breath, and blood sugar nightmare that it leaves behind. Staying off coffee will be a lifelong battle for me, and possibly for you as well. Try to switch from coffee to green tea. Green tea won't stain your teeth and is much lower in caffeine. It's also good for you. The antioxidants in green tea may prevent heart disease and cancer, and some research shows that it may also promote weight loss.

SOUND SUPPLEMENTS

I don't come from a family of sleepers, and grew up thinking that more than 5 hours of sleep was a waste of my precious time. Now, my days are long and physically strenuous. Because of this, I had to find natural ways to supplement and fortify my body. With the help of my sister Bonnie, I researched Chinese herbs and other supplements, and now ingest an assortment of pills each day for increased energy, stamina, and immunity.

Most of us don't eat Soundly all the time, and processed foods simply don't provide us with the nutrition we need. Couple that with air pollution, work stress, and the rigors placed upon your body during your Sound Training program, and a few supplements become a must.

Although you should never live on shakes and bars, they often come in handy when you're in a nutritional pinch. When supermodel and actress James King was in Austin, Texas, to make a movie, she took along a stash of protein bars. She knew she could look to them when all the food provided consisted of fatty, processed lunchmeats.

Here are the nutritional supplements that are most important to building a Sound body.

Protein bars. There are three basic types of energy bars: high-carbohydrate bars, high-protein bars, and balance bars that contain a moderate amount of carbohydrate, fat, and protein. I very rarely recommend eating carbohydrate bars unless you're about to faint just before a workout or you're about to run a race or cycle a century. They're filled with empty calories. Protein bars can come in handy just after a workout and when you need a snack to tide you over.

When buying bars, look at the food label. The fat content should be less than 6 grams and the saturated fat less than 3 grams. The sodium should be less than 200 milligrams and the carbohydrate less than 5 grams. A few grams of fiber is great. Look for a bar with about 30 grams of protein. Any more and you're eating a meal, not a snack. My favorite bar brands include the Ultimate Low Carb Bar, Designer Low

Sound Dining Out

Some of my clients have paid me to go out to eat with them, asking me to show them the path to Sound nutrition heaven—the gates beyond which only the purest of proteins and carbohydrates are allowed admission.

First of all, don't show up with an empty stomach. When you're hungry, all foods look and sound delicious. Always have a small protein shake, a protein bar, or an apple to take the edge off. (This goes for grocery shopping as well.) A little food in your belly will make it less likely that you'll binge on caloric hors d'oeuvres.

Here's how to make sounder dining choices, from beverage to dessert.

Beverage. Water with lemon or lime is the best choice. But if you feel the need for alcohol, hold yourself to one drink and go for wine or hard alcohol on the rocks or with club soda. Stay away from any drink that comes with an umbrella. It probably contains more calories than your entire meal. It's not a good idea to drink on an empty stomach, so drink with your meal, not before.

Appetizer. If you're going to have one, go for a salad with the dressing on the side. Or, if there's a Sound protein choice—such as sushi-grade tuna—go for it.

Main course. Try to have a piece of protein with a vegetable. If you see any of the following words or phrases, there's danger ahead: "sautéed," "fried," "pan roasted," or "light cream sauce." If the dish comes with a sauce, order it on the side since sauces are usually loaded with sugar, salt, cheese, butter, oil, or cream. Eat a sensible portion size. For meat, eat a piece no larger than the size of your hand. Pay attention to your hunger instead of stuffing yourself. Eat slowly, and when you're full, stop eating.

Dessert. Share it with friends. Poached pears, baked apples, and other types of fruit are the best choices. Watch out for sorbets, which can be loaded with sugar.

Carb Bar, and one by EAS called Myoplex Low Carb.

Protein powders. I like to add protein powder to my fruit shakes, especially if I'm drinking the shake right after a workout. Made up of amino acids, protein supplies the building blocks for your muscle growth. You could eat "real" protein after your workouts, such as a hard-boiled egg or some roasted turkey. But I've found that most people have trouble cooking three meals a day. They don't want to hit the kitchen for their snacks as well. (Also, it's better to have a mix of protein and carbohydrate rather than pure protein.)

At the health food store, you'll find various types of protein powders, from whey to soy to egg protein. Whey protein comes from milk protein minus the fat and sugar, and I prefer it to other types because your body absorbs it most efficiently. The brand Designer Protein contains 100 percent whey protein powder. You can find it at most local vitamin shops and health food stores, and it goes a long way toward replenishing your muscles and energizing your body.

Having a protein shake made with whey protein powder after your workouts will help you build muscle faster, speed your recovery time from your workout, reduce injuries and soreness, and generally help you enjoy your workouts more. Because protein breaks down slowly, a shake is great to have when you're hungry or before heading to a party or restaurant when you feel you might overindulge. Pre–cocktail party protein shakes would definitely be the number one answer given in a health-related version of *Family Feud*.

Amino acid supplements. For clients who have trouble eating the amount of food they need to help put on muscle, I often recommend taking branched-chain amino acids. These protein supplements won't fill you up, but they will give you the protein boost you need to put on the muscle that you want.

Mushrooms. Clients have told me that numerous types of exotic mushrooms—maitake, reishi, and shiitake—have boosted their energy levels during those first few weeks of the program when they were feeling tired. In addition to providing extra energy, some of these mushrooms also have antiviral and anticancer properties. They also may reduce blood pressure, blood cholesterol, and blood sugar levels, making them an overall Sound supplement choice. You can take these mushrooms once a day as a supplement, following the package directions. I recommend the brand Solaray.

Ginseng. One of the best energy boosters around, ginseng can also help boost your immunity and overall wellness. Because Korean ginseng can increase appetite, avoid it if you are trying to lose weight. Also, it has estrogenic properties, so don't use if you're a woman with hormone imbalances. Don't take either form of ginseng with caffeine, or you may feel jittery. Also, don't take it if you have hypertension or a heart condition. Follow the package directions.

Sound Mind, Sound Body Success Story

Before I started training at the Madison Square Club, I had been traveling for 4 months. I often entertained clients late at night with huge meals that included wine and dessert. During those 4 months, I gained 30 pounds.

I tried every trainer imaginable to help me get back in shape, but just wasn't seeing results. Then I found David. He told me to eliminate starchy carbs such as rice, pasta, bread, and processed foods. My body reacted to that, and the results were immediate. He took off 20 of those 30 pounds in the first 2 months.

I had been eating five meals a day and I was never hungry. Just eliminating those carbs and stepping up the intensity of my workouts really made a difference.

I've always used food as an emotional crutch, and I can't say I don't ever have a craving. I don't miss bread or pasta, but I do miss sugar every once in a while. Every time I crave those chocolate-chip cookies, I remember David's words: "You work too hard at looking and feeling a certain way to screw it up by eating this." That's usually all it takes to prevent me from overdoing it. And if I do have a bad day—or even a bad week—I just get myself back on track with a little discipline and a lot of David.

—Stephanie Fray

Glucosamine. One of the major building blocks of your body's cartilage, glucosamine reduces the joint pain that accompanies arthritis. It's a great supplement for those who avoid exercise because of knee or back pain. Take it before your workouts, and follow the package instructions.

Glutamine. An amino acid, glutamine is highly concentrated in your muscles. Taking it in supplement form can help you put on muscle, boost your immunity, and reduce soreness. Don't take glutamine if you have kidney or liver problems, if you are pregnant, or if you are breastfeeding. Take it before and after your workouts and follow the package instructions.

Astragalus. This Chinese herb can boost your immunity, preventing the colds and flu that can sometimes hinder your workouts. Because it's rich in polysaccharides, it increases the activity of numerous types of immune cells. Follow the package directions.

Vitamins A, C, and E; selenium; and coenzyme Q$_{10}$. These powerful antioxidants lend their electrons to

(continued on page 158)

The Sound Eating Quiz

It's time to work on your choice-making skills. Read through the following scenarios and pick what you think is the best choice. Then read on for some surprising answers.

Breakfast Choices

1. a) Fast-food breakfast sandwich
   b) Nonfat bran muffin
   c) Scrambled eggs with toast
   Few nonfat bran muffins are truly made from whole grains. And even fewer aren't loaded with sugar, salt, and calories. Most people know that those fast-food breakfast sandwiches are loaded with artery-clogging saturated fat. That leaves the scrambled eggs as your best choice.

2. a) Whole wheat pancakes with syrup
   b) Granola
   c) Special K with fat-free milk and artificial sweatener
   Granola is simply refined oatmeal that's been combined with gobs of honey, sugar, and oil, among other fattening ingredients. If the whole wheat pancakes were truly whole wheat (few are), and if they came along with some form of protein—they might create the best choice. The Special K—though I'm not thrilled about the artificial sweetener—provides the most balanced meal.

3. a) Fresh-squeezed fruit juice blend
   b) Fruit-flavored yogurt
   c) Bowl of fresh tropical fruit

Although tropical fruit and fruit juice are both good for your health, neither will keep hunger at bay all morning and both, without some protein, will send your blood sugar for a roller-coaster ride. For the yogurt, the best type is plain nonfat mixed with your own assortment of fresh berries. The "fruit" in fruit-flavored yogurt is mostly sugar.

Lunch Choices

4. a) Subway turkey sub on harvest wheat
   b) Big Mac
   c) Filet-O-Fish
   The Filet-O-Fish is both deep-fat fried as well as made from processed fish, the same stuff in fish sticks. The Subway turkey sub advertises that it contains fewer than 400 calories, but just about everything on it is either processed or of poor nutritional quality. Surprise! I'm going with the Big Mac, providing you hold the special sauce and cheese and ask them not to grill the bun.

5. a) Pasta primavera with vegetables
   b) Slice of pizza
   c) Mu shu chicken
   Far from a balanced meal, the pasta primavera provides 100 percent carbohydrate. Though pizza is not the worst food in the world (especially if you go light on the cheese), the best choice is actually the mu shu chicken, assuming you ask for it pre-

pared with steamed cabbage and Chinese vegetables, without the oil, and with white-meat chicken. Get the plum sauce—which is full of sugar—on the side, and hold yourself to one pancake.

6. a) Chef's salad
    b) Tuna salad on whole wheat
    c) Minestrone soup

This is a toss-up between the chef's salad and the tuna, depending on how they are prepared. A chef's salad with roasted turkey, roast beef, and hard-boiled egg whites is great. One with processed lunch meat is not. Tuna salad with big chunks of tuna, lots of veggies, very little mayo, served open-faced on only one slice of whole grain bread is also a good choice. (If you make tuna at home, wash the tuna first to get rid of the salt and other preservatives.) The minestrone comes with white pasta, white potatoes, and carrots—all on the unsound list for carbohydrates. It also contains no protein.

Dinner Choices

7. a) Spaghetti and meatballs
    b) Filet mignon with steamed spinach
    c) Shrimp Parmesan

None of these choices will win an award for soundest food choice of the year. Your best choice in this scenario is the filet mignon, assuming you go with the petite 6-ounce serving. By now you know what's wrong with spaghetti and meatballs. And the shrimp Parmesan contains fatty cheese and oil. Plus the shrimp is usually breaded and fried.

8. a) Fried chicken
    b) Baby back ribs
    c) Spaghetti bolognese

Both fried chicken and baby back ribs will set you back days for your intake of saturated fat. Surprise again! I'm going with the pasta. The meat in the bolognese sauce balances out this meal, and the tomato sauce adds some nutrition. It's easy to go overboard with pasta, so if you're at a restaurant, portion it so that you eat only two fistfuls worth.

9. a) Low-calorie frozen dinner
    b) Garden burger
    c) Rotisserie chicken

I'm not a big fan of low-calorie frozen dinners. While they may be low in calories, they're also low in nutrition and high in preservatives and salt. While touted as the health food of the 1990s, the garden burger probably contains more rice, refined grains, and oils than it does vegetables and soy protein. (Check the label to be sure.) That leaves you with the rotisserie chicken. Try to buy one that's free-range and organic. Go for the breast and leave the skin on your plate.

(continued)

The Sound Eating Quiz (cont.)

Daytime Snack Choices

10. a) Cheese and crackers
    b) Popcorn
    c) Almonds
    Even though popcorn has earned a repu-
    tation as the all-you-can-eat-and-not-get-
    fat binge food, I've yet to meet one person
    who felt energized after eating it. The
    cheese and crackers is slightly better. But
    the best choice is the nuts, which give you
    a dose of healthy omega-3 fats as well as
    some protein. Make sure to buy them raw,
    not roasted.

11. a) Frozen yogurt
    b) Rice cakes with jam
    c) Power Bar
    Fifteen minutes after eating your carb-
    laden rice cakes, you'll be hungry for
    more. Most energy bars contain more
    calories and carbohydrate than most
    people bargain for. That leaves the frozen
    yogurt.

12. a) Baby carrots
    b) Apple
    c) Grapes
    Because of their high sugar content, few
    people can stop at just a few grapes. Car-
    rots provide similar dissatisfaction, which
    brings us to the apple. Low on the
    glycemic index and at only 80 calories, it's
    an easy winner.

Nighttime Snack Choices

13. a) Peanut butter
    b) Low-fat ice cream
    c) Fat-free cookie
    I'd prefer you didn't snack at all at night,
    but if you're going to, make it protein. The
    fat-free cookie is all sugar. Same with the
    low-fat ice cream. Go with a teaspoon of
    peanut butter, especially if it's the natural
    type.

14. a) Baked potato chips
    b) Banana
    c) Yogurt
    Neither the banana nor the chips will sat-
    isfy your snacking urge, so go with the yo-
    gurt, the only option that contains some
    protein.

15. a) Chocolate bar
    b) Weight Watchers diet cheesecake
    c) Chocolate-covered strawberry
    The diet cheesecake is sweetened with
    fake sugar. And the chocolate bar is a
    binge waiting to happen. The chocolate-
    dipped strawberry will give you the sweet-
    ness you crave for a fraction of the
    calories.

Preworkout snack choices

16. a) Apple
    b) Pretzels
    c) "Light" candy bar
    Candy bars should be an obvious no-no. While the pretzels will supply your body with energizing and easily digestible carbohydrate for your workout, they give you little in the way of nutrition, leaving the apple as the best choice.

17. a) Baked potato
    b) Protein shake
    c) Balance Bar
    The protein shake and the Balance Bar wouldn't be bad choices at a different time of day. But just before a workout, their protein and fat will slow digestion. This is one of the few times when I'll tell you to go for the potato.

18. a) Fruit shake
    b) Turkey sandwich
    c) Beef jerky
    The protein in the turkey sandwich and beef jerky will slow digestion, and the salt in both of those cured products will bloat you. Go with the fruit shake.

Postworkout snack choices

19. a) Myoplex shake
    b) Whey protein shake
    c) Soy protein shake
    You need quality, lean protein within 45 minutes of your workout to help your muscles rebuild, and all three products will give you that protein. But the Myoplex shake will give you way too much—as well as some carbohydrate—turning your postworkout snack into a heavy postworkout meal. The soy shake isn't a bad choice, but your body will better absorb the whey protein shake.

20. a) High-protein bar
    b) High-carbohydrate bar
    c) Balance Bar
    The high-carbohydrate bar won't give you the protein you need. The Balance Bar isn't a terrible choice, but a high-protein bar is the best of the bunch.

21. a) Glass of milk
    b) Hard-boiled egg
    c) Orange
    While an orange might taste great right after a hot workout, it won't supply you with protein. The glass of milk contains some protein, but it also contains the milk sugar lactose. The hard-boiled egg provides the most absorbable protein choice of the three.

What to Eat, and When

You have a 6:00 P.M. workout and it's 5:00 P.M. You're so hungry that even the New York City street vendor's choices look like gourmet food. What to eat? a) candy bar b) apple or c) protein shake? If you chose (a), then we have a lot of work ahead of us. Although (c) might not seem like a bad choice, b) is definitely the more correct between the two.

At 7:00 P.M., however, after your workout, the protein shake would win out over the apple. You see, the best food choice changes depending on the circumstances and the time of day. The following 24-hour schedule of Sound Eating will help you better understand what to eat—and when to eat it.

6:00 A.M. to 9:00 A.M. Eat breakfast. It's a cliché, but it's true. Breakfast is the most important meal of the day. Don't skip it. Make your breakfast high in protein, as this will help get you through the morning hunger-free. Good choices include eggs, turkey sausage, and yogurt. If you're the type of person who needs some carbohydrate, try some fresh fruit or oatmeal (minus the sugar, raisins, and cream.)

10:30 A.M. If you're starving, have a low-carbohydrate snack such as a little yogurt. If you're not hungry mid-morning, skip the snack.

Noon to 2:00 P.M. Eat lunch. Make this a balanced meal that includes a Sound protein source such as chicken or fish and Sound carbohydrate such as a salad. A little bit of healthy fat from nuts or olive oil is fine.

4:30 P.M. Have some Sound carbohydrate such as a side of steamed broccoli or spinach or an apple.

free radicals in your body, making them more stable and preventing them from destroying other cells. In turn, this can prevent a host of problems from general aging to heart disease to cancer to arthritis and even to cataracts. Your best defense against free radicals is multilevel, and that's why I suggest various antioxidant supplements rather than just one.

You can get all of these antioxidants, plus a dose of other helpful vitamins and minerals from the multiple vitamin and mineral supplement Solaray VM 2000. I recommend taking vitamin E and selenium as separate supplements since vitamin C can lower your absorption of them.

Milk thistle. This herb enhances the metabolism of your liver cells,

5:00 P.M. to 8:00 P.M. Eat dinner. Make your dinner a balanced meal with a Sound protein choice and a Sound carbohydrate choice with a little bit of fat. For example, have sesame-encrusted salmon with a side of asparagus.

9:00 P.M. to 6:00 A.M. This is the RED ZONE. Eating during this time tends to be mood-related, not hunger-related. Try to get in control of what's driving you to the cupboard, fridge, or freezer. If you need to eat something, make it high in protein. When I'm craving food late at night, I have a teaspoon of all-natural peanut butter. It stops the cravings every time.

Your Sound Eating choices will be slightly different depending on your body type. (For more on body types, see page 116.)

If you're an apple, pear, or round type and are trying to lose weight, you should never eat in the RED ZONE. Try to make your food choices as pure as possible, especially the carbohydrate choices, and try not to snack during the morning.

If you're a stick trying to gain weight, protein shakes are a must. You need to eat a lot of food, probably more than you feel comfortable eating. Three square meals are a must, as well as two or three snacks. Have a protein shake after your workout, and another just before bedtime. You're the only body type that's allowed to eat in the red zone. Take an amino acid supplement as well as some Korean ginseng to boost your appetite.

If you're the fit type, you'll find that you'll see more definition if you cut out starchy carbs and slightly increase your protein intake.

protecting them from toxins. It's a great detoxification herb. Follow the package directions.

Garlic. A natural antiseptic and antibiotic, garlic has been shown to lower blood cholesterol levels. To avoid bad garlic breath, opt for deodorized tablets.

Cranberry extract. Just like cranberry juice but without the calories, this supplement helps flush out your kidneys. Follow the package directions.

Flaxseed oil. Sold in capsules or in liquid form, this oil contains the important omega-3 fatty acids I mentioned earlier. It has been known to make those with the most stubborn constitutions become rather regular. (Don't try flaxseed oil for the first time on the day of a new date.)

EATING RIGHT FOR WORKING OUT

Your eating schedule will change slightly depending on the time of day you work out. If you are fueling up before a workout, you want something that's easy to digest. That's where carbohydrates come in. That's the best time to have those sugary snacks that I've warned you against. (Of course, an apple or other type of quality carbohydrate would be a better choice.) After your workout, you need protein to help your muscles rebuild themselves.

With that in mind, here are some sample schedules for different workout times.

THE MORNING WORKOUT

I love morning workouts because the body is most conducive to lifting weights between 7:30 and 10:30 A.M. In fact, when I was a practicing attorney, my workouts started at 5:00 A.M.

Try to work out on an empty stomach, as this will help you burn fat. If you must, have ½ cup of tea or coffee and a nibble of food such as an apple. Just don't eat anything too heavy.

Note: If you take morning medications, you'll have to eat to help your body best absorb the medication. Also, if it's the weekend and you're working out after 10:00 A.M., you'll need to eat breakfast before your ex-

ercise session. Make sure to get out of bed 90 minutes before your workout to have a fruit shake or some other easy-to-prepare high-carbohydrate meal.

Immediately after your morning workout, have a protein snack such as a protein shake or yogurt with berries.

One hour later, after you've showered and dressed for work, have a high-protein breakfast such as an egg and vegetable omelette. If you're on the run and don't have time for a sit-down breakfast, turn that post-workout shake into a meal by adding two scoops (2 tablespoons) of protein powder rather than just one. That will give you about 36 grams of protein, depending on the type of protein used.

THE MIDDAY WORKOUT

For workouts between noon and 2:00 P.M., you don't need a preworkout snack unless you are starving. In that case, just have a few bites from an apple.

After your workout, have a protein shake, hit the showers, get dressed, and then eat a nice protein lunch with veggies at your desk.

If you're working out later in the afternoon, say 3:00 P.M., you'll need to change your strategy somewhat. Make sure to eat a light lunch before 1:00 P.M.; if your lunch is too heavy, you'll want to nap instead of work out. For example, I would stay away from steak for lunch. Following your

David's Indispensable Kitchen List

Although this list is not meant to be comprehensive, these are some of the things I could not live without in my kitchen. And neither should you.

◆ Food processor or blender

◆ An assortment of nonstick pans and skillets

◆ Steaming basket

◆ Salad spinner

◆ A good set of knives—make sure to keep them clean and frequently sharpened

◆ Healthy supply of your favorite mustards (Dijon, whole grain, and flavored). Check the ingredients for the sugar content—try to keep it as low as possible. And just FYI—honey is sugar in disguise.

◆ Vinegars, including, balsamic, red wine, white wine, rice, and flavored

◆ Salt and pepper mills for that fresh-ground salt and pepper taste

◆ Nonfat vegetable cooking spray

◆ Horseradish, wasabi, Tabasco, and any other of your favorite hot and spicy sauces

◆ Homemade or low-fat, low-sodium chicken broth. If homemade, I like to store and freeze the broth in ice trays.

◆ Fresh roasted garlic paste (can be made ahead and frozen)

◆ Oven-roasted tomatoes (can be made ahead and frozen)

◆ Roasted red peppers (can be made ahead and frozen)

◆ Nonfat plain yogurt—This will be used in place of mayonnaise and in some dressings. Stick with the plain variety, as the fruited yogurts often add fruit preserves which are much more dense in sugars.

◆ Fresh strawberries and blueberries washed, trimmed, and frozen

◆ Fresh produce—At the Madison Square Club, we like to prewash greens and store them for days in advance.

◆ Fresh herbs—Fresh herbs are best preserved by keeping them in fresh water covered loosely in plastic until ready to use. Stored this way, they will last all week. Cut off what you need, wash and dry it, then prepare it for use. (For emergency purposes, always have a good supply of dried herbs on hand.)

workout, you'll need a protein shake or other protein snack to carry you through until dinnertime.

THE EVENING WORKOUT

If you're hitting the gym right after work, you'll need a light carbohydrate snack at 4:00 P.M. to give you energy during your workout. The snack should be easily digestible, such as an apple, pear, potato, half an energy bar, or a small fruit drink. After your workout, eat a protein snack, especially if you'll be having dinner at a restaurant or party where you'll be tempted to drink alcohol. A protein shake with a half-scoop (3 teaspoons) of protein after your workout will help coat your stomach, preventing you from stuffing yourself silly with alcohol and food.

If you're working out even later at night, such as 8:00 or 9:00 P.M., you'll need to eat a light dinner beforehand. Unless you're as thin as a "stick," avoid eating after 9:00 P.M. That's the red zone. Rearrange your day so that lunch is your largest meal and dinner is more of a snack than a meal. Don't misunderstand me; you need to eat

dinner, but the Italians definitely have it right with a larger lunch and a lighter dinner.

SOUND = SIMPLE

Whether working out or preparing food, the philosophy is the same in my Sound Mind, Sound Body formula—less is more. That said, the relative simplicity of the recipes on the following pages should not mislead anyone into thinking that these foods aren't loaded with flavor.

At the Madison Square Club, we've found that the key to eating Soundly is in creating exceptional flavors with the fewest ingredients. And when possible, adding a bit of zip. Feel free to make substitutions where necessary or desired, and experiment with herbs, flavor boosters, or special ingredient combinations that are exclusively your own. Note that many of the recipes call for bottled water. You will find that this is an essential ingredient since you are limited in the types of liquid you should use.

Sound Cooking Secrets

Steaming Vegetables

The healthiest way to prepare cooked vegetables is to steam them over simmering water. A steamer basket is essential for this purpose. For the most flavor, add 1 teaspoon Madison Square Club Herb Blend (page 166) and 1 teaspoon of your favorite herbed vinegar to the steaming water before bringing to a boil. Or, replace half of the steaming water with Chicken Stock (page 164)

Peeling and Seeding Tomatoes

When a recipe calls for diced tomatoes, I prefer to use peeled, seeded tomatoes. The extra flavor is worth the extra effort.

To peel: Make an X with a knife on the bottom of the tomato. Drop it into a pot of boiling water for 30 seconds. Remove the tomato and place it in an ice water bath. Immediately slip off the tomato peel with your fingertips or a paring knife.

To seed: Cut the tomato in half and scoop out the seeds with a small spoon.

Handling Hot Peppers

Many of our dishes call for jalapeño, serrano, and other hot peppers. Here are a few pointers that I learned the hard way:

◆ If possible, use gloves when handling hot peppers. If you can't use gloves, take care not to touch the seeds or the cut surfaces of the pepper, which contain the searing heat. Using two utensils can help you avoid touching the pepper with your hands while cutting it.

◆ When finished handling hot peppers, discard the gloves and thoroughly wash the knife and cutting board.

◆ Unless you want your food to be blisteringly hot, use only the flesh of the pepper and discard the seeds.

Julienning Herbs

Salads, entrées, and soups all look more appetizing with a garnish of julienned large-leaf herbs such as basil or mint. To julienne large-leaf herbs, stack the leaves, then roll them up like a cigar. Slice crosswise across the cigar to make thin strips.

BASICS

Some of the recipes that follow call for prepared items like chicken stock, roasted peppers, or dried tomatoes. In most cases, you can use store-bought versions, but you'll get better flavor by making them yourself. Here are instructions for making some basic items that I like to keep on hand.

CHICKEN STOCK

This recipe is an MVP in my kitchen. From sauces to steaming, it more than earns its keep.

1 whole, bone-in chicken (3 pounds)
4 quarts cold bottled water
1 Vidalia onion, chopped
2 celery ribs, greens included, chopped
2 spring onions or scallions, chopped
1 tablespoon Roasted Garlic Paste (opposite page) or 1 garlic clove, minced
1 bunch parsley
4–5 sprigs fresh thyme or 1 teaspoon dried
1 tablespoon tricolor peppercorns or 2 teaspoons fresh coarsely ground black pepper
1 bay leaf

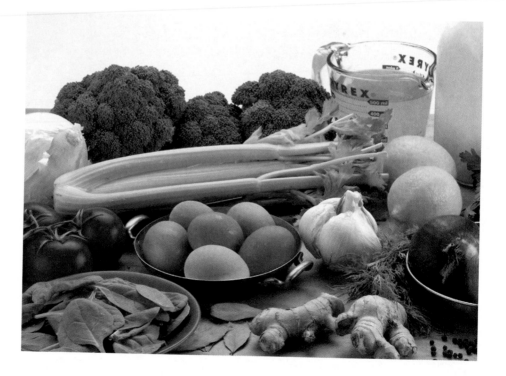

Wash and cut the chicken into pieces at the joints (or have your butcher do it). Place the chicken in a large stockpot. Add the water and bring to a boil over high heat. Skim any foam that rises to the surface.

Add the Vidalia onion, celery, spring onions or scallions, and garlic. Return to a boil, then immediately reduce the heat to medium-low. Gently simmer for 2 hours, uncovered, skimming the foam occasionally and adding more water if necessary to keep the chicken submerged.

Add the parsley, thyme, peppercorns or black pepper, and bay leaf. Simmer for 1 hour more.

Strain the stock through a sieve, pressing the solids to extract the liquid. Discard the solids. Pull the chicken meat off the bones and reserve for another use. Let the stock cool to room temperature, then refrigerate until cold. Remove and discard the fat that congeals on surface. Pour the stock into ice cube trays and freeze until solid. Transfer the cubes to freezer bags and freeze for up to 3 months. *Makes 12 servings. Per serving: 10 calories, 0 g protein, 2 g carbohydrate, 0 g fat, 0 g saturated fat, 1 g fiber, 1 g sugar*

POACHED CHICKEN BREAST

You can also use this recipe to poach other foods, such as fish. The poaching times may vary, but the results are delicious.

1   **cup bottled water**
1   **cup Chicken Stock (opposite page) or low-fat, low-sodium chicken broth**
1   **tablespoon tricolor peppercorns**
4   **ounces boneless, skinless chicken breast**

Pour the water and stock into a stockpot or deep sauté pan. Bring to a gentle boil and add the peppercorns and chicken, making sure the chicken is totally covered by liquid. (Add more water or stock if necessary.) Reduce the heat to a simmer. Cook for about 12 minutes, until the chicken is fork-tender and is no longer pink. Avoid overcooking, which will dry out the chicken. *Makes 1 serving. Per serving: 130 calories, 27 g protein, 0 g carbohydrate, 1 g fat, 0 g saturated fat, 0 g fiber, 0 g sugar*

ROASTED GARLIC PASTE

I love the sweet and subtle flavor of roasted garlic. I like to roast and puree lots of it, then freeze it so I can keep it on hand in place of raw garlic.

3   **heads of garlic**

Preheat the oven to 350°F. Remove any loose, papery skin from the garlic. Place the whole garlic head on a baking dish or in a clay roaster. Cover tightly with foil or the lid of the roaster. Bake for 1 hour, until the garlic is soft. Let cool while still covered. Peel and discard the skin.

Puree the garlic in a food processor and drop in 1-tablespoon portions onto a foil-lined baking sheet. Freeze until solid, then store in an airtight plastic bag until ready to use. *Makes 8 servings. Per serving: 13 calories, 1 g protein, 3 g carbohydrate, 0 g fat, 0 g saturated fat, 0 g fiber, 0 g sugar*

OVEN-DRIED TOMATOES

2   small plum tomatoes
1   tablespoon balsamic vinegar

Preheat the oven to 250°F. Coat a baking sheet with cooking spray. Thinly slice the tomatoes lengthwise into 6 or 7 slices and arrange on the baking sheet. Drizzle with the vinegar and bake for 1½ hours. Remove from the oven and let cool. Use within 1 day or freeze in an airtight plastic bag until ready to use. When ready to use, remove the tomatoes from the freezer and use as is. Or, if you want them crispy, bake at 250°F for a few minutes. *Makes 2 servings. Per serving: 18 calories, 1 g protein, 4 g carbohydrate, 0 g fat, 0 g saturated fat, 1 g fiber, 3 g sugar*

MADISON SQUARE CLUB HERB BLEND

1   tablespoon chopped fresh dill
1   tablespoon chopped fresh parsley
1   tablespoon chopped fresh basil
1½   teaspoons chopped fresh thyme

Mix the herbs and use immediately. Or refrigerate for up to 3 hours before using. *Makes 4 servings. Per serving: 1 calories, 0 g protein, 0 g carbohydrate, 0 g fat, 0 g saturated fat, 0 g fiber, 0 g sugar*

ROASTED RED PEPPERS

3   red bell peppers (or use yellow, orange, or green)

Preheat the broiler. Cut off the tops of the peppers. Remove the core and seeds from each. Cut the peppers lengthwise into quarters. Lay the pieces skin side up on a baking pan. Broil until the skin is charred. Remove from the heat. When cool enough to handle, remove and discard the skin using a paring knife. Use immediately or freeze in an airtight plastic bag for up to 3 weeks. *Makes 3 servings. Per serving: 44 calories, 1 g protein, 11 g carbohydrate, 0 g fat, 0 g saturated fat, 3 g fiber, 4 g sugar*

EGGS AND BREAKFAST DISHES

CLASSIC EGG-WHITE OMELETTE

At the Madison Square Club, egg-white omelettes are our favorite way to start the day. They're easy to make, low in fat, and satisfying. And the variations are endless. Here's the classic egg-white omelette. Use this to get started, then add your own market-fresh ingredients. Use whatever vegetables are in season. If you like a slightly richer omelette, add 1 egg yolk to the white.

- 3 egg whites
- 1 tablespoon fat-free milk
  Freshly ground black pepper
- 1 tablespoon finely chopped fresh herbs such as chives, parsley, and marjoram

Heat a 9" nonstick skillet over medium-high heat and coat with cooking spray.

In a small bowl, whisk together egg whites and milk. Season to taste with the pepper. Add the egg mixture to the skillet and sprinkle with the herbs. Cook for about 30 seconds, or until the edges begin to brown. Do not overcook. Using a spatula, loosen the edges, then fold the omelette in half. Invert onto a serving plate. *Makes 1 serving. Per serving: 57 calories, 11 g protein, 2 g carbohydrate, 0 g fat, 0 g saturated fat, 0 g fiber, 2 g sugar*

ASPARAGUS FRITTATA

Frittatas are great for a crowd. We love to make our asparagus frittata for spring brunch. In summer, try sweet tomatoes and basil instead of the asparagus. Or try sautéed shiitake mushrooms with garlic or steamed broccoli.

- 11 egg whites
- 1 whole egg
- ¼ cup fat-free milk
  Salt and pepper
- 1 cup asparagus, trimmed, steamed, and cut into 1" pieces (see page 163)

Preheat the oven to 350°F. In a medium bowl, whisk together the egg whites, whole egg, and milk. Season to taste with the salt and pepper. Pour into a 9" round ovenproof baking dish. Arrange the asparagus pieces evenly over the egg mixture. Bake for 25 to 30 minutes, until center is just set. Do not overbake. Let cool for 2 to 3 minutes. Cut into wedges and serve. *Makes 6 servings. Per serving: 52 calories, 8 g protein, 2 g carbohydrate, 1 g fat, 0 g saturated fat, 0 g fiber, 2 g sugar*

THE MSC BREAKFAST WRAP

Definitely beats those fast-food breakfast sandwiches, and has a lot less fat!

- 1 piece Armenian flatbread, cut into quarters
- 8 strips natural (nitrate-free) turkey bacon
- 12 egg whites
- 4 tablespoons fat-free milk
  Freshly ground black pepper

Preheat oven to 250°F. Wrap each slice of flatbread in foil. Place in the oven to warm.

In a nonstick skillet, cook the bacon over medium heat for 4 to 6 minutes, until browned on both sides. Remove to paper towels, blot, and set aside.

In a small bowl, whisk together the egg whites and milk. Season to taste with the pepper. Set aside.

Wipe out the skillet and heat over medium-high heat. Coat with cooking spray. Add the egg mixture and cook for about 2 minutes, stirring occasionally, until just set. Remove the flatbread pieces from the oven. Arrange 2 bacon slices and one-quarter of the egg mixture on each piece of flatbread. Roll the bread around the filling and serve immediately. *Makes 4 servings. Per serving: 207 calories, 18 g protein, 19 g carbohydrate, 6 g fat, 2 g saturated fat, 1 g fiber, 3 g sugar*

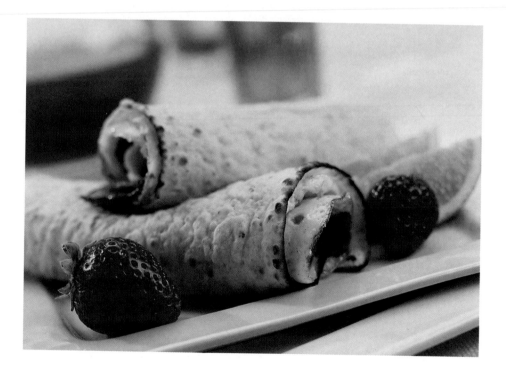

HUEVOS RANCHEROS

A healthy Mexican breakfast may seem like an oxymoron, but here at the club, anything is possible.

- ¼ cup sliced Vidalia onions
- ¼ cup sliced red and/or yellow bell peppers
- 4 egg whites
- 1 tablespoon fat-free milk
- 1 tablespoon bottled water
  Salt and pepper
  Chopped parsley, for garnish

Heat a medium nonstick skillet over medium-high heat and coat with cooking spray. Add the onion and bell pepper. Cook for 3 minutes, stirring often, until softened. Set aside and keep warm.

In a small bowl, whisk together the egg whites, milk, and water. Season to taste with the salt and pepper. Pour into the skillet used to cook the vegetables and cook for 3 to 4 minutes, until set. Once set, flip the eggs and place the onion and bell pepper mixture in the center. Garnish with the parsley and serve immediately. *Makes 1 serving. Per serving: 93 calories, 15 g protein, 7 g carbohydrate, 0 g fat, 0 g saturated fat, 1 g fiber, 5 g sugar*

SAUCES AND DRESSINGS

SPICY PEANUT SAUCE

Finally, a peanut sauce without the coconut milk or added sugar. Try this on poached chicken or as a dip for fresh vegetables.

- ¼ cup unsweetened peanut butter
- ¼ cup bottled water
- 2 tablespoons fresh lime juice
- 1 tablespoon low-sodium soy sauce
- ½ teaspoon grated lime zest
- ½ teaspoon minced garlic or 1 teaspoon Roasted Garlic Paste (page 165)
- ½ teaspoon grated fresh gingerroot
- ½ teaspoon Thai chili paste

In a small bowl or food processor, combine the peanut butter, water, lime juice, soy sauce, lime zest, garlic, ginger, and chili paste. Mix until smooth. Use immediately or refrigerate for up to 3 days. *Makes 10 servings. Per serving: 40 calories, 2 g protein, 2 g carbohydrate, 3 g fat, 0 g saturated fat, 0 g fiber, 1 g sugar*

FAT-FREE HORSERADISH CREAM SAUCE

Whether on broiled trout or poached salmon, this sauce tastes like the "Ultimate Cheat." Try it on steamed vegetables, too.

- ¼ cup nonfat plain yogurt
- 1 tablespoon white horseradish
- ¼ teaspoon minced garlic
- ¼ teaspoon ground white pepper

In a small bowl or food processor, combine the yogurt, horseradish, garlic, and pepper. Mix until smooth. *Makes 5 servings. Per serving: 8 calories, 1 g protein, 2 g carbohydrate, 0 g fat, 0 g saturated fat, 0 g fiber, 1 g sugar*

SUMMER SALSA

Great spooned over grilled fish or chicken.

- ¼ cup diced mango
- ¼ cup diced papaya
- ¼ cup coarsely chopped orange sections
- ¼ cup diced cantaloupe
- ¼ cup chopped red onion
  Juice of 1 lime
- 1 tablespoon chopped fresh parsley
- 1 teaspoon chopped jalapeño pepper (optional)

In a medium bowl, mix the mango, papaya, orange, cantaloupe, onion, lime juice, parsley, and jalapeño pepper (if using). Refrigerate for at least 1 hour before serving. *Makes 8 servings. Per serving: 14 calories, 0 g protein, 4 g carbohydrate, 0 g fat, 0 g saturated fat, 0 g fiber, 2 g sugar*

BALSAMIC VINAIGRETTE

This is the classic fat-free dressing at the Madison Square Club. We use it as a base for countless dressing variations. Here's the basic recipe with 4 variations.

- ¼ cup balsamic vinegar
- 2 tablespoons bottled water
- 1 tablespoon lemon juice
- 1 teaspoon Dijon mustard
- 1 teaspoon honey
  Fresh ground black pepper

In a small bowl or glass jar, combine the vinegar, water, lemon juice, mustard, and honey. Season to taste with the pepper. Whisk or shake until mixed. Use immediately or refrigerate for up to 1 week. *Makes 8 servings. Per serving: 9 calories, 0 g protein, 2 g carbohydrate, 0 g fat, 0 g saturated fat, 0 g fiber, 2 g sugar*

VARIATIONS

Ginger-Balsamic Dressing: Add 1 teaspoon grated fresh gingerroot and 3 or 4 drops of sesame oil along with the vinegar.

Lemon Burst Vinaigrette: Add 1 tablespoon minced shallot and ½ teaspoon grated lemon zest along with the vinegar.

Herb Balsamic Vinaigrette: Add 1 tablespoon chopped fresh herbs (such as 1 teaspoon thyme, 1 teaspoon dill, and 1 teaspoon parsley) along with the vinegar.

Strawberry Vinaigrette: Puree 2 frozen strawberries and 1 tablespoon bottled water. Add the strawberry mixture to the vinaigrette along with the vinegar.

CITRUS CILANTRO DRESSING

Fresh and clean-tasting, this dressing is wonderful on Tuna Salad Niçoise (page 174). Try it on salads, too.

- 2 tablespoons fresh orange juice
- 1 tablespoon bottled water
- 2 teaspoons fresh lime juice
- 2 teaspoons fresh lemon juice
- 1 teaspoon whole grain mustard
- ½ teaspoon grated orange zest
- ½ teaspoon chopped cilantro
- ½ teaspoon olive oil (optional)

In a small bowl or glass jar, combine the orange juice, water, lime juice, lemon juice, mustard, orange zest, cilantro, and oil (if using). Whisk or shake until mixed. Use immediately or refrigerate for up to 1 week. *Makes 5 servings. Per serving: 6 calories, 0 g protein, 1 g carbohydrate, 0 g fat, 0 g saturated fat, 0 g fiber, 1 g sugar*

FAT-FREE RANCH DRESSING

The perfect partner for Cod Cakes (page 185).

- ½ cup nonfat plain yogurt
- 1 tablespoon Madison Square Club Herb Blend (page 166)
- 1 teaspoon finely chopped shallots
- 1 teaspoon Roasted Garlic Paste (page 165) or 1 clove garlic, minced
- 1 teaspoon capers, rinsed well, and chopped if large
- 1 teaspoon whole grain mustard

In a small bowl or glass jar, combine the yogurt, herb blend, shallots, garlic, capers, and mustard. Whisk or shake until mixed. Use immediately or refrigerate for up to 2 days. *Makes 10 servings. Per serving: 7 calories, 1 g protein, 1 g carbohydrate, 0 g fat, 0 g saturated fat, 0 g fiber, 1 g sugar*

GINGER SOY DRESSING

One of the more versatile dressings at the club. We use it on grilled chicken and Thai Ginger Sirloin Salad (page 172).

- 2 tablespoons rice wine vinegar
- 2 tablespoons bottled water
- 1 tablespoon low-sodium soy sauce
- 1 teaspoon sesame oil
- 1 teaspoon honey
- 1 teaspoon grated fresh gingerroot
- 1 teaspoon toasted sesame seeds

In a small bowl or glass jar, combine the vinegar, water, soy sauce, oil, honey, ginger, and sesame seeds. Whisk or shake until mixed. Use immediately or refrigerate for up to 1 week. *Makes 5 servings. Per serving: 32 calories, 0 g protein, 3 g carbohydrate, 1 g fat, 0 g saturated fat, 0 g fiber, 3 g sugar*

SALADS AND SOUPS

THAI GINGER SIRLOIN SALAD

Fabulous hot or cold. When chilled, the steak is not as spicy, so we use ½ teaspoon red-pepper flakes when serving this salad. If serving it warm, we use only ¼ teaspoon red-pepper flakes and the steak is still quite spicy. If baby bok choy is not available, use an extra cup of mesclun greens instead. The salad is a little less crunchy but still delicious.

6   ounces sirloin steak, trimmed of fat
1   teaspoon grated fresh gingerroot
1   clove garlic, minced
¼–½ teaspoon red-pepper flakes
    Juice of ½ lime
1   head baby bok choy cabbage, sliced (about 1 cup)
1   cup mesclun greens, washed and dried
1   tablespoon grated carrot
¼   cup bean sprouts
3   tablespoons Ginger Soy Dressing (page 171)

Cut the sirloin into ½" slices and place in a small bowl. Add the ginger, garlic, and pepper flakes. Squeeze the juice of ½ lime over the meat. Toss to coat. Let marinate at room temperature for 10 to 15 minutes.

Meanwhile, heat a medium nonstick skillet over medium-high heat and coat with cooking spray. Add the bok choy and cook for 1 to 2 minutes, until the leaves are just wilted but the cabbage is still crunchy. Remove to a serving plate.

Wipe out the skillet and coat with cooking spray. Heat over high heat. Place the sirloin slices in the pan and sear for 30 seconds per side for rare or 50 seconds per side for well-done. Set aside.

Line a serving plate with the bok choy, mesclun greens, carrot, and bean sprouts. Arrange the steak over the salad. Serve immediately or refrigerate for up to 6 hours and serve chilled. Drizzle with dressing just before serving. *Makes 1 serving. Per serving: 363 calories, 33 g protein, 18 g carbohydrate, 15 g fat, 5 g saturated fat, 3 g fiber, 9 g sugar*

VARIATION

Thai Ginger Tofu Salad: Replace the beef with 6 ounces firm tofu. Omit the lime juice from the marinade and use ⅛–¼ teaspoon red-pepper flakes. Sear the tofu for 15 seconds per side. We prefer the tofu when it has been just seared. If making ahead, set the tofu aside from the salad and toss together with dressing when ready to serve.

TOMATO SHALLOT SALAD

This salad is excellent topped with Sesame Salmon (page 187).

2   tablespoons fresh lime juice
1   tablespoon low-sodium soy sauce
1   tablespoon chopped fresh dill
½   teaspoon Dijon mustard
¾   cup quartered grape tomatoes
1   tablespoon chopped shallots

In a small bowl, whisk together the lime juice, soy sauce, dill, and mustard.

Add the tomatoes and shallots. Toss to coat. Spoon onto a serving plate. *Makes 1 serving. Per serving: 52 calories, 3 g protein, 11 g carbohydrate, 1 g fat, 0 g saturated fat, 1 g fiber, 1 g sugar*

Thai Ginger Sirloin Salad

QUINOA SALAD

Crunchy and delicious, this grain salad is rich in complete protein and calcium.

½ cup quinoa
1 cup bottled water
¼ cup diced cucumber
¼ cup peeled, seeded, and diced tomato
3 orange segments, chopped coarsely
2 tablespoons chopped celery
2 tablespoons Citrus Cilantro Dressing (page 171)
   Fresh cilantro leaves for garnish

Rinse and drain the quinoa in a fine mesh strainer under running tap water until the water runs clear.

Bring the water to a boil in a small saucepan. Add the quinoa and cook for 15 minutes over medium-low heat, until all of the water is absorbed.

Meanwhile, in a medium bowl, combine the cucumber, tomato, orange segments, celery, and dressing. Add quinoa and toss to mix. Refrigerate until cold. Garnish with cilantro leaves and serve chilled. *Makes 2 servings. Per serving: 179 calories, 6 g protein, 33 g carbohydrate, 3 g fat, 0 g saturated fat, 3 g fiber, 3 g sugar*

TUNA SALAD NIÇOISE

This French classic—minus the potatoes and egg yolks—gets a flavor makeover with our tangy Citrus Cilantro Dressing.

4 ounces Romaine lettuce leaves, washed and dried and torn into pieces
2 spears asparagus, steamed and cut into 1" pieces
1 ounce haricot verts or thin green beans, trimmed and steamed (about 8 pieces)
4 grape tomatoes, halved
¼ cup peeled, cubed jicama
1 tablespoon chopped chervil
1 tablespoon chopped chives
4 ounces sushi-grade (Grade A) tuna steak
   Salt and pepper
1 hard-cooked egg white, quartered
2 tablespoons Citrus Cilantro Dressing (page 171)

In a medium bowl, combine the lettuce, asparagus, haricot verts or green beans, tomatoes, jicama, chervil, and chives. Arrange on a serving plate.

Season the tuna steak with salt and pepper. Heat a grill pan over high heat and coat with cooking spray. Add the tuna and cook for 1 minute. Turn and cook 1 to 2 minutes more, until seared on the outside but still rare in the center. Slice the tuna steak into ½" slices and arrange with the egg white over the salad. Drizzle with the dressing. Serve immediately. *Makes 1 serving. Per serving: 212 calories, 35 g protein, 15 g carbohydrate, 2 g fat, 0 g saturated fat, 6 g fiber, 3 g sugar*

SPICY THAI SHRIMP SALAD

Tastes great grilled, too. Once marinated, skewer the shrimp and grill for 1 to 2 minutes per side.

- 3 jumbo shrimp, peeled and deveined
- 2 slices lemon, coarsely chopped
- 1 clove garlic, minced
- 1 teaspoon grated fresh gingerroot
- ¼ teaspoon red-pepper flakes
- ⅛ teaspoon salt
- 2 cups washed, dried, and shredded Romaine lettuce leaves
- 1 scallion, sliced
- 3 basil leaves, julienned (see page 163)
- 3 tablespoons Spicy Peanut Sauce (page 169)

"Butterfly" each shrimp by slicing it lengthwise without cutting through to the other side, then flattening it on your work surface.

In a small bowl, combine the butterflied shrimp, lemon, garlic, ginger, red-pepper flakes, and salt. Toss to coat. Cover and refrigerate for 1 hour to marinate.

Heat a medium nonstick skillet over high heat and coat with cooking spray. Add the shrimp and cook over high heat for 2 minutes per side, until cooked through. Set aside.

Arrange the lettuce, scallion, and basil on a serving plate. Top with the shrimp and drizzle with the peanut sauce. Serve immediately or at room temperature. *Makes 1 serving. Per serving: 170 calories, 12 g protein, 11 g carbohydrate, 9 g fat, 2 g saturated fat, 5 g fiber, 4 g sugar*

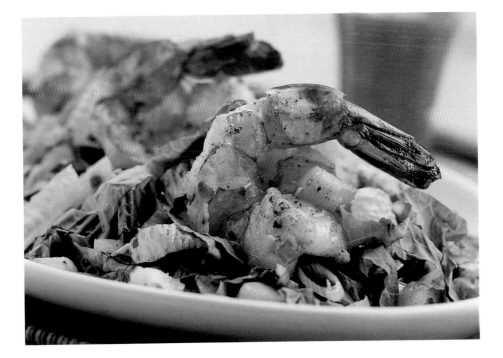

CHICKPEA SALAD WITH SALSA FRESCA

A classic Middle Eastern dish goes South of the Border.

- 1 cup cooked or canned chickpeas, rinsed well
- 1 plum tomato, peeled, seeded, and coarsely chopped (see page 163)
- ¼ cup chopped sweet red onion
- ¼ cup chopped Roasted Red Pepper (page 166)
- 2 tablespoons apple cider vinegar
- 1 tablespoon chopped fresh cilantro
- 1 tablespoon chopped jalapeño pepper

  Salt and pepper

In a medium bowl, combine the chickpeas, tomato, onion, roasted red pepper, vinegar, cilantro, and jalapeño pepper. Season to taste with the salt and black pepper. *Makes 1 serving. Per serving: 264 calories, 10 g protein, 53 g carbohydrate, 3 g fat, 0 g saturated fat, 10 g fiber, 15 g sugar*

CUCUMBER SALAD

This is one of our standard summer recipes at the club. Its versatility lends itself to many combinations. We like to serve it alongside Chicken Satay (page 184).

- 1 cup thinly sliced seedless cucumber
- ¼ cup thinly sliced red onion
- 2 tablespoons rice wine vinegar
- ¼ teaspoon red-pepper flakes

In a small bowl, combine the cucumber, onion, vinegar, and pepper flakes. Toss to mix. Cover and refrigerate or set aside at room temperature for 2 to 3 hours before serving to allow the flavors to blend. *Makes 1 serving. Per serving: 98 calories, 1 g protein, 16 g carbohydrate, 0 g fat, 0 g saturated fat, 2 g fiber, 12 g sugar*

CHICKEN PAPAYA SALAD

Just a hint of papaya turns this otherwise ordinary low-calorie dish into a tropical feast. To make this dish ahead, combine all the salad ingredients minus the dressing, then cover and refrigerate for up to 8 hours. Toss with dressing when ready to serve.

- 4 ounces Poached Chicken Breast, diced (page 165)
- 2 cups baby spinach leaves, washed and dried
- ½ cup sliced endive, washed and dried
- ¼ cup diced papaya (2 ounces)
- 2 tablespoons diced red onion
- 2 tablespoons diced fennel bulb
- 2 tablespoons store-bought fat-free lemon–poppy seed yogurt dressing

In a medium bowl, combine the chicken, spinach, endive, papaya, onion, fennel, and dressing. Toss to mix. Arrange on a serving plate and serve immediately. *Makes 1 serving. Per serving: 228 calories, 36 g protein, 12 g carbohydrate, 4 g fat, 1 g saturated fat, 3 g fiber, 6 g sugar*

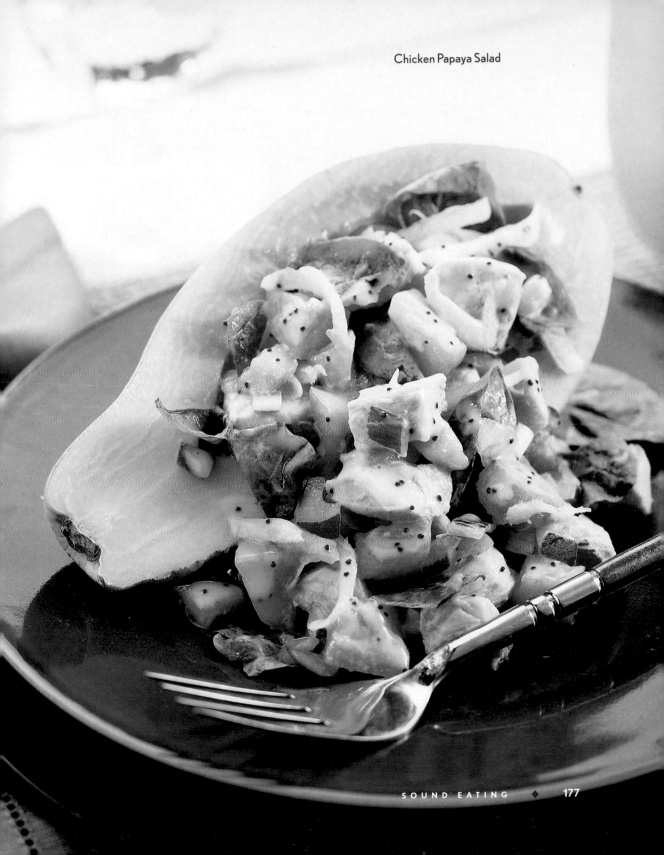

Chicken Papaya Salad

COUSCOUS SALAD

Simply delicious. I use it alongside main-dish salads or fish entrees.

- ½ cup cooked couscous
- 1½ tablespoons nonfat plain yogurt
- 1 tablespoon minced green bell pepper
- 1 tablespoon diced tomato
- 1 tablespoon minced scallion
- 1 teaspoon chopped fresh parsley
- ¼ teaspoon grated lemon zest
  Fresh ground black pepper

In a medium bowl, combine the couscous, yogurt, bell pepper, tomato, scallion, parsley, and lemon zest. Season to taste with the black pepper. Serve immediately or refrigerate for up to 1 day. *Makes 1 serving. Per serving: 106 calories, 4 g protein, 22 g carbohydrate, 0 g fat, 0 g saturated fat, 2 g fiber, 2 g sugar*

ROASTED TURKEY BASIL SALAD

You can use any sliced fresh turkey breast, but we like to use leftovers from Herb-Crusted Turkey Breast (page 184).

- 2 tablespoons chopped fresh basil
- 1 tablespoon chopped fresh parsley
- 6 ounces sliced roasted turkey breast
- 2½ cups Romaine lettuce leaves, cleaned and torn into pieces
- 3 grapefruit sections
- 2 tablespoons Fat-Free Ranch Dressing

Place the basil leaves and parsley in a medium bowl. Mash into a chunky paste with the back of a spoon, adding a few drops of water if necessary.

Add the turkey and toss to coat. Line a serving plate with the lettuce. Arrange the turkey and grapefruit on top. Drizzle with the dressing just before serving. *Makes 1 serving. Per serving: 337 calories, 55 g protein, 25 g carbohydrate, 2 g fat, 0 g saturated fat, 5 g fiber, 11 g sugar*

GAZPACHO

For a more complete meal, I sometimes add 2 grilled shrimp to each serving. Top this soup with plenty of fresh dill.

- 2 large ripe tomatoes, cored
- 1 red bell pepper, cored, seeded, and chopped
- 1 yellow bell pepper, cored, seeded, and chopped
- 1 cucumber, peeled, seeded, and chopped
- ½ cup chopped Pomi tomato
- ¼ cup red wine vinegar
- 1 jalapeño pepper, seeded and chopped (see page 163)
- 1 tablespoon Madison Square Club Herb Blend (page 166)
  Salt and pepper
- ½ red onion, chopped, for garnish

In a blender or food processor, combine the ripe tomatoes, half of the red bell pepper, half of the yellow bell pepper, and half of the cucumber. Blend until slightly chunky. Transfer to a large bowl and add the Pomi tomato, vinegar, jalapeño pepper, herb blend, and remaining bell pepper and cucumber. Season to taste with the salt and pepper. Garnish with the red onion. *Makes 1 serving. Per serving: 160 calories, 6 g protein, 36 g carbohydrate, 2 g fat, 0 g saturated fat, 9 g fiber, 14 g sugar*

BLACK BEAN–ROASTED RED PEPPER SOUP

A hearty, stick-to-your-ribs soup that'll leave you feeling satisfied and nourished.

⅔ cup dried black beans
½ cup finely chopped onion
¼ cup diced celery
1 clove garlic, minced
1 quart bottled water
1 bay leaf
½ teaspoon dried thyme leaves
¼ teaspoon ground cumin
⅛ teaspoon red-pepper flakes
⅓ cup diced Roasted Red Pepper (page 166)
1 tablespoon chopped fresh parsley
Salt and pepper

Soak the beans overnight in enough water to generously cover. Drain and set aside.

Heat a 2-quart saucepan over medium-high heat and coat with cooking spray. Add the onion, celery, and garlic, and cook for 3 to 5 minutes, until softened. Add the beans, water, bay leaf, thyme, cumin, and pepper flakes. Bring to a boil. Reduce heat to medium-low and simmer gently for 30 minutes. Add the roasted red pepper and parsley. Cook for another 15 to 20 minutes, until the beans are soft and the soup is thick. Add more water if the soup is too thick. Season to taste with the salt and pepper. Remove and discard the bay leaf before serving. *Makes 2 servings. Per serving: 224 calories, 14g protein, 43 g carbohydrate, 1 g fat, 0 g saturated fat, 13 g fiber, 3 g sugar*

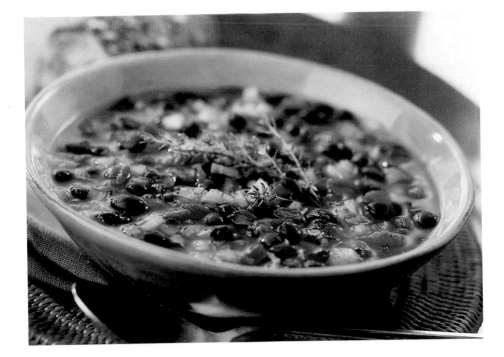

HONEYDEW TOMATILLO SOUP

Light and refreshing, this soup makes a good first course. Or add ¼ cup fresh crabmeat for a more complete meal.

½	cup chopped tomatillos (2 to 3 large)
1	cup cubed honeydew melon
1–2	teaspoons chopped jalapeño pepper
1	teaspoon chopped fresh parsley
¼	cup finely diced honeydew
¼	cup fresh crabmeat (optional)
1	scallion, thinly sliced
4	mint leaves, julienned (see page 163)

In a blender or food processor, combine the tomatillos, melon, jalapeño pepper, and parsley. Blend until pureed. Cover and refrigerate. Just before serving, garnish with the diced honeydew, crabmeat (if using), scallion, and mint. *Makes 1 serving. Per serving: 109 calories, 2 g protein, 26 g carbohydrate, 1 g fat, 0 g saturated fat, 3 g fiber, 20 g sugar*

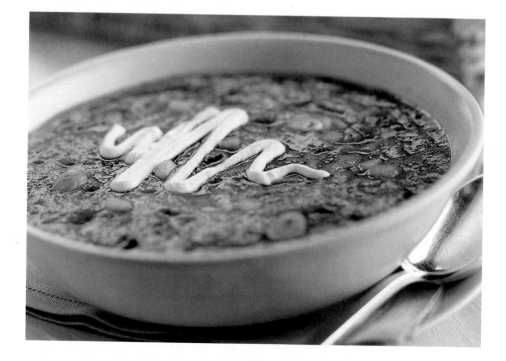

MAIN DISHES

TURKEY MEATBALLS WITH SPAGHETTI SQUASH MARINARA

This is the second most popular dish at the Madison Square Club. I like to serve this entrée with cooked greens such as spinach or kale.

1	spaghetti squash (4–5 pounds)
1	Vidalia onion, chopped
1	clove garlic, minced
6	plum tomatoes, chopped
½	cup chopped Pomi tomatoes
2	tablespoons low-sodium tomato paste
½	cup fresh basil leaves, finely chopped
¾	pound lean ground turkey
1	egg white
2	tablespoons finely chopped shallots
1	tablespoon Dijon mustard
1	tablespoon chopped fresh parsley
1	teaspoon chopped fresh oregano
⅛	teaspoon freshly ground black pepper
2–3	dashes hot-pepper sauce

Preheat the oven to 400°F. Wrap the whole squash in foil. Place it on a baking sheet and bake for 1 to 1½ hours, until tender when pierced with a fork, turning the squash over halfway through cooking. Set aside to cool.

Heat a medium nonstick skillet over medium heat and coat with cooking spray. Add the onions and garlic and cook for 2 to 3 minutes, until softened. Add the plum tomatoes, Pomi tomatoes, tomato paste, and basil. Simmer gently for 15 minutes. Set aside.

In a medium bowl, combine the turkey, egg white, shallots, mustard, parsley, oregano, pepper, and hot-pepper sauce. Mix gently and shape into 8 meatballs.

Heat a large nonstick skillet over medium-high heat and coat with cooking spray. Add the meatballs and cook for 4 to 5 minutes, turning often, until browned all over. Pour the marinara sauce over the meatballs in the skillet. Cover and simmer for 8 to 10 minutes, until the meatballs are cooked through.

Cut the cooked spaghetti squash in half. Remove and discard the seeds. Scoop out 3 cups of squash from the shell. (Reserve the remaining squash for future use.) Arrange the squash on a serving platter and top with the meatball–marinara sauce mixture. *Makes 2 servings. Per serving: 483 calories, 38 g protein, 48 g carbohydrate, 18 g fat, 4 g saturated fat, 11 g fiber, 12 g sugar*

VARIATION

Buffalo Meatballs with Spaghetti Squash Marinara: Replace the turkey with ground buffalo meat for a higher-protein, richer-tasting meatball. Buffalo is leaner and has a much bolder flavor. Cook the buffalo meatballs for 6 to 8 minutes to be sure they are fully browned.

TURKEY CHILI

The all-time favorite at the Madison Square Club. If you like thick chili, cook it longer or stir in 1 tablespoon unsweetened peanut butter. For spicier chili, increase the cayenne to ¼ teaspoon.

1 pound lean ground turkey
  Salt and pepper
2 carrots, peeled and grated (1 cup)
1 onion, chopped (¾ cup)
2 ribs celery, chopped (⅔ cup)
1 clove garlic, minced
2 teaspoons chili powder
1 teaspoon paprika
1 teaspoon ground cumin
⅛ teaspoon ground cayenne pepper
1 can (14½ ounces) chopped plum tomatoes in juice
½ cup Chicken Stock (page 164) or low-fat, low-sodium chicken broth
1 bay leaf

Heat a 3-quart nonstick saucepan over high heat and coat with cooking spray. Add the turkey and season to taste with the salt and pepper. Cook for 2 to 3 minutes, breaking up the turkey into pieces, until browned all over. Remove to a bowl and cover with foil to keep warm.

Reduce the heat to low and add the carrots, onion, celery, and garlic. Cook for 3 to 5 minutes, until the vegetables begin to soften. Add the chili powder, paprika, cumin, and cayenne pepper. Cook, stirring, for 1 minute. Increase the heat to medium and add the tomatoes, stock, and bay leaf. Bring to a boil over high heat. Reduce the heat to medium-low and simmer for 15 minutes, uncovered.

Add the browned turkey and simmer for 5 minutes more. Remove and discard the bay leaf before serving. *Makes 4 servings. Per serving: 240 calories, 23 g protein, 15 g carbohydrate, 10 g fat, 3 g saturated fat, 4 g fiber, 8 g sugar*

TURKEY MEAT LOAF

Serve with steamed spinach and Cauliflower Hash (page 191). For a more bold-flavored meatloaf, replace the turkey with ground buffalo.

½ cup chopped onion
¼ cup chopped celery
¼ cup chopped carrot
½ teaspoon paprika
½ teaspoon salt
⅛ teaspoon ground cayenne pepper
⅛ teaspoon freshly ground black pepper
8 ounces lean ground turkey
1 egg white
¾ cup diced canned plum tomatoes in juice

Preheat the oven to 350°F. Heat a medium nonstick skillet over medium heat and coat with cooking spray. Add the onion, celery, and carrot. Cook for 3 minutes, until softened. Stir in the paprika, salt, cayenne pepper, and black pepper. Cook for 1 minute. Remove to a medium bowl and let cool for 2 minutes.

Add the turkey, egg white, and tomatoes to the bowl. Mix until just blended. Shape into a loaf and place in an ovenproof baking dish or loaf pan. Bake for 30 to 40 minutes, until no longer pink in the center and a thermometer inserted registers 165°F. *Makes 2 servings. Per serving: 232 calories, 23 g protein, 12 g carbohydrate, 10 g fat, 3 g saturated fat, 2 g fiber, 8 g sugar*

Turkey Chili

HERB-CRUSTED TURKEY BREAST

The secret is using plenty of fresh herbs and whole grain mustard. We like to make this turkey breast for dinner, then use the fresh roasted turkey for salads. The herb crust and relatively low roasting temperature guarantee moist turkey. As you remove the skin before serving, sprinkle the turkey with chopped fresh parsley and coarse black pepper. Serve with pureed cauliflower and steamed spinach for a healthy traditional meal.

2 tablespoons chopped fresh thyme
2 tablespoons Dijon mustard
1 tablespoon chopped fresh oregano
1 teaspoon chopped fresh rosemary
½ teaspoon freshly ground black pepper
1 whole turkey breast (4–5 pounds)

Preheat the oven to 350°F.

In a small bowl, combine the thyme, mustard, oregano, rosemary, and pepper. Place the turkey breast in a roasting pan, skin side up. Spread the herb mixture evenly over the top. Bake for 1¼ to 1½ hours, until juices run clear and a thermometer inserted in the thickest portion registers 170°F. Remove and discard the skin before serving. *Makes 6 servings. Per serving: 212 calories, 46 g protein, 1 g carbohydrate, 2 g fat, 0 g saturated fat, 0 g fiber, 0 g sugar*

Chicken Satay and Cucumber Salad (p. 176)

CHICKEN SATAY

With the spices and the peanut sauce, you'll feel like you've been transported to Thailand. Serve with Cucumber Salad (page 176).

6 ounces boneless, skinless chicken breast
½ teaspoon curry powder
¼ teaspoon ground cayenne pepper
⅛ teaspoon freshly ground black pepper
3 tablespoons Spicy Peanut Sauce (page 169)

Slice the chicken into 6 pieces and place in a small bowl. Add the curry powder, cayenne pepper, and black pepper. Toss to coat. Cover and refrigerate for 1 to 2 hours to marinate.

Preheat the broiler or grill. Thread the chicken onto skewers and broil or grill 4" from the heat for 2 to 3 minutes per side, until no longer pink. Serve with peanut sauce. *Makes 1 serving. Per serving: 312 calories, 46 g protein, 7 g carbohydrate, 11 g fat, 3 g saturated fat, 2 g fiber, 2 g sugar*

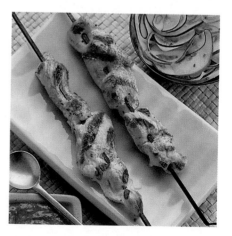

SHIITAKE CHICKEN PAILLARD

6 ounces boneless, skinless chicken breast
  Salt and pepper
¾ cup sliced shiitake mushrooms (2 ounces)
1 clove garlic, minced
2 tablespoons balsamic vinegar
¼ cup Chicken Stock (page 164) or low-fat, low-sodium chicken broth
1 teaspoon chopped fresh thyme

Place the chicken between sheets of plastic and pound with a meat mallet to ⅛" thickness. Season both sides of the chicken with the salt and pepper.

Heat a large nonstick skillet over medium-high heat and coat with cooking spray. Place the chicken on one side of the heated pan. Place the mushrooms and garlic on other side. Cook the chicken for 2 minutes, until browned. Turn and cook for 3 minutes, until the chicken is no longer pink. While the chicken is cooking, cook the mushrooms and garlic for 3 to 4 minutes, until lightly browned. Remove the chicken and mushroom mixture to a serving plate.

Add the balsamic vinegar, stock, and thyme to the pan. Bring to boil over high heat. Reduce the heat to medium-low and simmer for 30 seconds, until slightly thickened. Pour over the chicken and serve immediately. *Makes 1 serving. Per serving: 231 calories, 42 g protein, 9 g carbohydrate, 2 g fat, 1 g saturated fat, 1 g fiber, 5 g sugar*

COD CAKES

I like to add 2 tablespoons of chopped cornichons (tiny pickles) to the dressing for extra zip.

5 ounces cod fillet
⅓ cup chopped Vidalia onion
⅓ cup diced Roasted Red Pepper (page 166)
1 egg white
1 tablespoon chopped fresh parsley
1 teaspoon chopped fresh dill
⅛ teaspoon salt
⅛ teaspoon freshly ground black pepper
1 cup mesclun greens
2 tablespoons Fat-Free Ranch Dressing (page 171)

Preheat the oven to 400°F. Coat a 1½-quart baking dish with cooking spray. Arrange the cod in the dish and bake for 10 to 12 minutes, until the fish flakes easily when tested with a fork. Set aside to cool.

Heat a medium nonstick skillet over medium heat and coat with cooking spray. Add the onions and cook for 3 minutes, until just softened. Transfer to a medium bowl. Using a fork, flake the cod into the bowl. Add the roasted red pepper, egg white, parsley, dill, salt, and black pepper. Stir to mix. Shape into 4 patties.

Wipe out the skillet and heat over high heat. Coat with cooking spray. Add the cod cakes and cook for 1 to 2 minutes, until just browned on one side. Turn and cook for 1 to 2 minutes more, until just browned on the other side.

Line a serving plate with the mesclun greens. Top with the cod cakes and drizzle with the dressing. *Makes 1 serving. Per serving: 170 calories, 30 g protein, 9 g carbohydrate, 1 g fat, 0 g saturated fat, 2 g fiber, 4 g sugar*

ALMOND-CRUSTED CATFISH

The almonds jive up this recipe with crunchy texture and taste as well as additional calcium. I like to serve this with Quinoa Salad (page 174) and Ginger Soy Dressing (page 171).

6 ounces farm-raised catfish fillet
   Salt and freshly ground black pepper
1 tablespoon blanched chopped almonds
3 slices Oven-Dried Tomato, coarsely chopped (page 166)
2 cups broccoli rabe or spinach, trimmed and steamed
1 tablespoon Herb Balsamic Vinaigrette (page 170)

Season the catfish to taste with the salt and pepper. Press the chopped almonds into the top of the fillet.

Heat a large nonstick skillet over high heat and coat with cooking spray. Place the catfish, almond side down, into the hot pan. Reduce the heat to medium and cook for about 2 minutes, until browned. Turn and cook for 2 to 3 minutes more, until fish just flakes easily when tested with a fork.

In a small bowl, toss the tomato with the broccoli rabe or spinach. Arrange on a serving plate and top with the catfish. Drizzle with the vinaigrette. *Makes 1 serving. Per serving: 348 calories, 34 g protein, 14 g carbohydrate, 18 g fat, 3 g saturated fat, 2 g fiber, 3 g sugar*

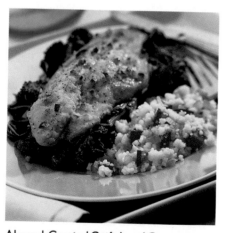

Almond-Crusted Catfish and Couscous Salad (p. 178)

ROASTED CHILEAN SEA BASS WITH VIDALIA ONIONS AND SUMMER SQUASH

1 Vidalia onion, sliced (1 cup)
½ cup julienned yellow squash
½ cup julienned zucchini squash
1 teaspoon chopped summer savory
6 ounces Chilean sea bass fillet
   Salt and pepper

Preheat the oven to 400°F. Heat a medium nonstick skillet over medium-low heat and coat with cooking spray. Add the onion and cook for 15 to 20 minutes, until very soft and slightly caramelized. Reduce the heat to low if the onions begin to burn. Add the squash and summer savory. Raise the heat to high and cook for 2 to 3 minutes. Remove to a 1½-quart baking dish.

Place the sea bass on the vegetables and sprinkle with the salt and pepper. Bake for 15 to 20 minutes, until the fish just flakes easily when tested with a fork. *Makes 1 serving. Per serving: 251 calories, 35 g protein, 20 g carbohydrate, 4 g fat, 1 g saturated fat, 6 g fiber, 11 g sugar*

SESAME SALMON

My personal favorite. It's crunchy on the outside, versatile, and easy to make. At the club, we pair it with 1 cup steamed broccoli rabe in winter or Tomato Shallot Salad (page 172) in summer. We also use a mixture of black and white sesame seeds. But white seeds alone work just as well.

6   ounces salmon fillet
    Salt and pepper
2   teaspoons sesame seeds

Season the salmon to taste with the salt and pepper. Press the seeds into the top of the fillet to make a crust. Heat a large nonstick skillet over high heat and coat with cooking spray. Place the salmon in the pan with the sesame seeds down. Cook for 2 minutes, until the sesame seed crust is golden brown. Using a spatula, carefully turn the salmon and cook for 2 to 3 minutes more, until the salmon is just opaque throughout. *Makes 1 serving. Per serving: 346 calories, 35 g protein, 1 g carbohydrate, 21 g fat, 4 g saturated fat, 1 g fiber, 0 g sugar*

SEARED TUNA WITH SPICY WASABI SLAW

1   tablespoon rice wine vinegar
1   tablespoon water
1   teaspoon low-sodium soy sauce
½   teaspoon grated wasabi root
½   teaspoon grated fresh gingerroot
⅛   teaspoon sesame oil or 2 teaspoons toasted sesame seeds
½   cup snow pea shoots
½   cup julienned daikon radish (see page 163)
1   scallion, sliced
2   tablespoons grated carrot
6   ounces sushi-grade (Grade A) tuna steak
2   teaspoons freshly ground black pepper

In a medium bowl, whisk together the vinegar, water, soy sauce, wasabi, ginger, and sesame oil or seeds. Add the snow pea shoots, radish, scallion, and carrot. Toss to mix.

Heat a 9" nonstick skillet over high heat and coat with cooking spray. Coat both sides of the tuna with the pepper. When the pan is very hot, place the tuna in the pan and cook for 30 seconds over high heat to sear. Turn the tuna and cook for 30 seconds more to sear the other side. Arrange the slaw on a serving plate and top with the tuna. *Makes 1 serving. Per serving: 280 calories, 42 g protein, 16 g carbohydrate, 3 g fat, 1 g saturated fat, 4 g fiber, 9 g sugar*

GRILLED TUNA STEAK WITH ARUGULA AND VIDALIA ONIONS

This recipe can be made on a grill or in a grill pan. If you are grilling, place the onions on the grill as well.

½ Vidalia onion, thinly sliced (½ cup)
2 cups arugula, trimmed and washed
Salt and pepper
½ lemon
6 ounces sushi-grade (Grade A) tuna steak

Heat a small nonstick skillet over low heat and coat with cooking spray. Add the onions and cook for 10 to 12 minutes, until very soft. Raise the heat to high and cook for 1 minute, stirring, until the onions begin to brown. Add the arugula and cook for 1 minute. Sprinkle with the salt, pepper, and lemon juice. Transfer to a serving plate.

Preheat the grill or heat a grill pan over high heat and coat with cooking spray. Season both sides of the tuna with the salt and pepper. Place on the grill or in the pan and cook for 1 minute, until seared. Turn and cook for 1 to 2 minutes more, until other side is seared yet the tuna is still rare in the center. Place on top of the arugula mixture and serve. *Makes 1 serving. Per serving: 227 calories, 40 g protein, 12 g carbohydrate, 2 g fat, 1 g saturated fat, 2 g fiber, 6 g sugar*

OVEN-ROASTED HALIBUT NIÇOISE

A summer favorite at the club. We like to serve it over 2 cups mesclun greens tossed with 2 ounces steamed haricot verts (or thin green beans) and 3 tablespoons Balsamic Vinaigrette (page 170).

6 ounces halibut steak
1 teaspoon capers, chopped if large
1 teaspoon red wine vinegar
1 teaspoon chopped fresh thyme
2 Kalamata olives, pitted and chopped
½ teaspoon minced garlic
⅛ teaspoon freshly ground black pepper

Preheat the oven to 375°F. Place the halibut in a 1-quart baking dish.

In a small bowl, combine the capers, vinegar, thyme, olives, garlic, and pepper. Spread the mixture on top of the halibut, pressing firmly to make an even crust. Bake for 25 to 30 minutes, until fish just flakes easily when tested with a fork. *Makes 1 serving. Per serving: 206 calories, 36 g protein, 3 g carbohydrate, 5 g fat, 1 g saturated fat, 1 g fiber, 0 g sugar*

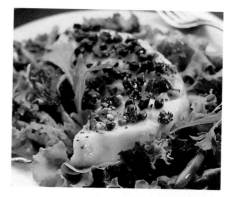

Oven-Roasted Halibut Niçoise

SIDE DISHES

NO-FAT HUMMUS

For more zip, add more cayenne pepper or a few drops of hot-pepper sauce.

1½   cups cooked or canned chickpeas, rinsed
¼   cup nonfat plain yogurt
1   tablespoon chopped parsley
1   teaspoon minced garlic
¼   teaspoon ground cumin
¼   teaspoon ground cayenne pepper
¼   cup fresh-squeezed lemon juice

In a food processor, combine the chickpeas, yogurt, parsley, garlic, cumin, cayenne pepper, and lemon juice. Process until well blended. Use immediately or refrigerate for up to 3 days. *Makes 2 servings. Per serving: 227 calories, 12 g protein, 40 g carbohydrate, 3 g fat, 0 g saturated fat, 10 g fiber, 4 g sugar*

CAULIFLOWER MUSHROOM MASH

One of the most popular side dishes at the club. It looks, feels, and almost tastes like mashed potatoes—minus all the carbs. Perfect with Turkey Meat Loaf (page 182) and other hearty main dishes.

½   cup sliced mushrooms
1   tablespoon chopped shallots
1   cup steamed cauliflower florets
1   teaspoon whole grain mustard
1   tablespoon chopped fresh parsley
    Freshly ground black pepper

Heat a small nonstick skillet over high heat and coat with cooking spray. Add the mushrooms and shallots, and cook for 2 to 3 minutes over high heat. Transfer to a food processor and let cool slightly. Add the cauliflower and mustard, and puree until smooth. If the mixture is too thick, add 1 to 2 tablespoons water. Stir in the chopped parsley and pepper. *Makes 1 serving. Per serving: 58 calories, 4 g protein, 10 g carbohydrate, 1 g fat, 0 g saturated fat, 5 g fiber, 3 g sugar*

ROASTED VEGETABLE CAPONATA

1 medium eggplant
½ cup chopped Vidalia onion
½ cup chopped fennel bulb
¼ cup chopped celery
1 clove garlic, minced
⅓ cup diced roasted red pepper
4 canned plum tomatoes, chopped
½ cup juice from canned tomatoes
½ cup bottled water
1 tablespoon coarsely chopped fresh parsley
4 fresh basil leaves
2 teaspoons baby capers (optional)

Preheat the oven to 400°F. Wrap the eggplant in foil and bake for 50 to 60 minutes, until tender when pricked with a fork. Cut the eggplant in half and scoop out 1 cup roasted eggplant from center. Set aside. (Reserve the remaining eggplant for future use.)

Heat a medium nonstick skillet over medium heat and coat with cooking spray. Add the onions and cook for 3 to 4 minutes, until they begin to soften. Add the fennel, celery, and garlic, and cook for 3 minutes. Add the roasted eggplant, roasted red pepper, plum tomatoes, juice, water, parsley, and basil. Simmer for 15 to 20 minutes, until the liquid is absorbed and the vegetables are soft. Remove the basil leaves and add the capers (if using). Remove from the heat and cool to room temperature. Cover and refrigerate for up to 2 weeks. Serve at room temperature. *Makes 2 servings. Per serving: 86 calories, 3 g protein, 20 g carbohydrate, 1 g fat, 0 g saturated fat, 5 g fiber, 10 g sugar*

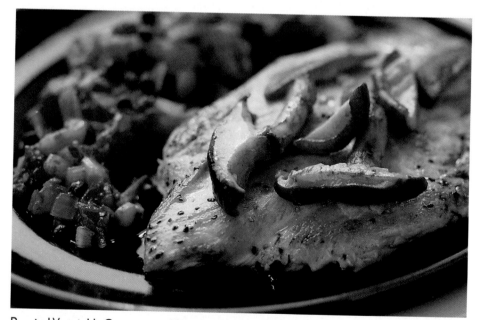

Roasted Vegetable Caponata and Shiitake Chicken Paillard (p. 185)

CAULIFLOWER HASH

I sometimes add 1 cup Herb-Crusted Turkey Breast (page 184) or cubed grilled chicken to make an entrée. For a vegetarian entrée, serve over steamed spinach.

- ¼ cup chopped shallots
- 1 cup cauliflower florets, steamed (see page 163)
- ⅓ cup chopped celery
- ⅓ cup diced Roasted Red Pepper (page 166)
- 1 teaspoon chopped fresh thyme
  Salt and pepper

Heat a medium nonstick skillet over medium heat and coat with cooking spray. Add the shallots and cook for 1 to 2 minutes, until softened. Add the cauliflower and celery. Cook for 3 to 5 minutes, until the vegetables begin to brown. Add the roasted red pepper and thyme. Cook for 2 minutes more. Season to taste with the salt and pepper. *Makes 2 servings. Per serving: 41 calories, 2 g protein, 9 g carbohydrate, 0 g fat, 0 g saturated fat, 2 g fiber, 2 g sugar*

ROASTED BRUSSELS SPROUTS

Excellent with Herb-Crusted Turkey Breast (page 184) and loaded with vitamin C and fiber.

- 1 cup halved brussels sprouts
- 1 teaspoon lemon juice
- 1 teaspoon minced chives
  Salt and pepper

Preheat the oven to 400°F. Place the brussels sprouts on a large piece of foil. Sprinkle with the lemon juice, chives, salt, and pepper. Fold up foil to enclose the ingredients and place on a baking sheet. Bake for 30 minutes, until the brussels sprouts are cooked through and lightly browned. Remove from the foil packet immediately and serve. *Makes 1 serving. Per serving: 39 calories, 3 g protein, 8 g carbohydrate, 0 g fat, 0 g saturated fat, 3 g fiber, 2 g sugar*

ASIAN BROCCOLI STIR-FRY

Works alongside most entrées. And it's a fabulous source of calcium and vitamin C.

- 2 cups broccoli florets, washed
- 1 clove garlic, minced
- 1 teaspoon grated gingerroot
- ¼ cup bottled water
- 2 teaspoons low-sodium soy sauce
- ⅛ teaspoon sesame oil

Heat a large nonstick skillet over high heat and coat with cooking spray. Add the broccoli and cook for 2 minutes, stirring. Add the garlic and ginger, and cook for 1 minute. Add the water, soy sauce, and sesame oil. Cover and cook for 2 to 3 minutes, until the broccoli is tender-crisp. *Makes 1 serving. Per serving: 59 calories, 5 g protein, 9 g carbohydrate, 1 g fat, 0 g saturated fat, 4 g fiber, 3 g sugar*

DESSERTS

SUNBURST BAKED APPLE WITH CINNAMON STICK

1   medium Rome or Cortland apple
1   cinnamon stick
¼   teaspoon lemon zest

Preheat the oven to 400°F. Partially core the apple (about ¾ of the way down to the blossom end). Place the cinnamon stick and lemon zest in the hole. Cover loosely with foil and bake for 30 minutes. Remove the foil and bake for 30 minutes more. Serve immediately. *Makes 1 serving. Per serving: 80 calories, 0 g protein, 22 g carbohydrate, 0 g fat, 0 g saturated fat, 5 g fiber, 16 g sugar*

CITRUS-MINT SALAD

1   orange, sectioned and juice reserved
1   blood orange, sectioned and juice reserved
1   pink grapefruit, sectioned
¼   cup reserved juice from orange and blood orange
½   vanilla bean, split
2   teaspoons chopped fresh mint

In a small bowl, combine the orange, blood orange, and grapefruit. Divide between two serving bowls.

In a small saucepan, combine the reserved liquid, vanilla bean, and mint. Bring to a boil over high heat. Reduce the heat to medium-low and simmer for 3 to 5 minutes, until liquid is reduced by half. Pour over the fruit and refrigerate for 1 to 2 hours. Serve chilled. *Makes 2 servings. Per serving: 111 calories, 2 g protein, 29 g carbohydrate, 0 g fat, 0 g saturated fat, 9 g fiber, 20 g sugar*

POACHED PEARS

1   Anjou pear, cut in half lengthwise, seeded, and peeled
¼   cup fresh-squeezed orange juice
¼   cup bottled water
½   orange, sliced with peel on
2   pieces star anise
¼   teaspoon whole coriander seeds
½   vanilla bean, split
6   raspberries
2   sprigs fresh mint

Place the pears in a medium saucepan. Add the orange juice, water, orange slices, star anise, coriander seeds, and vanilla bean (the liquid should partially cover the pears). Bring to a gentle simmer over medium-low heat. Do not let boil. Gently simmer for 15 to 20 minutes, until very tender. Carefully transfer to a shallow serving dish and pour the poaching liquid over top. Refrigerate until ready to use. Served cold or at room temperature garnished with raspberries and mint. *Makes 2 servings. Per serving: 95 calories, 1 g protein, 23 g carbohydrate, 1 g fat, 0 g saturated fat, 4 g fiber, 17 g sugar*

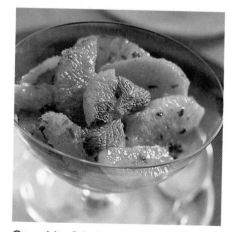

Citrus-Mint Salad

GREEN MELON
AND PARSLEY GRANITA

2   cups cubed green melon (Galia or
    honeydew)
2   teaspoons chopped fresh parsley
2   teaspoons fresh-squeezed lemon
    juice
½   teaspoon lemon zest

In a food processor, combine the melon, parsley, lemon juice, and lemon zest. Blend until pureed. Transfer to a small saucepan and cook over medium heat for 3 minutes, until slightly thickened. Transfer to a shallow airtight container and freeze until ready to use. Remove from the freezer 20 minutes before serving to soften. Scoop into serving dishes. *Makes 4 servings. Per serving: 32 calories, 0 g protein, 8 g carbohydrate, 0 g fat, 0 g saturated fat, 1 g fiber, 8 g sugar*

STRAWBERRY-RASPBERRY
GRANITA

1½ cups strawberries
1   cup raspberries
3   tablespoons orange juice
1   tablespoon lemon juice
1   teaspoon honey
½   teaspoon lemon zest

In a food processor, combine the strawberries, raspberries, orange juice, lemon juice, honey, and lemon zest. Blend until pureed. Transfer to a shallow airtight container and freeze until ready to use. Remove from the freezer 20 minutes before serving to soften. Scoop into serving dishes. *Makes 4 servings. Per serving: 44 calories, 1 g protein, 11 g carbohydrate, 0 g fat, 0 g saturated fat, 3 g fiber, 7 g sugar*

DRINKS

DAVID'S PLAIN AND SIMPLE
PROTEIN SHAKE

10 ounces mineral water
    (noncarbonated)
5   ice cubes
1   scoop vanilla Designer Protein
    powder

In a blender, combine the water, ice cubes, and protein powder. Blend on high speed for 45 seconds. Serve immediately. *Makes 1 serving. Per serving: 220 calories, 17 g protein, 35 g carbohydrate, 1 g fat, 0 g saturated fat, 1 g fiber, 27 g sugar*

PREWORKOUT
FRUIT SHAKE

8   ounces mineral water
    (noncarbonated)
5   ice cubes
¼   cup fresh blueberries, frozen
¼   cup fresh strawberries, frozen

In a blender, combine the water, ice cubes, blueberries, and strawberries. Blend on high speed for 45 seconds. Serve immediately. *Makes 1 serving. Per serving: 114 calories, 0 g protein, 29 g carbohydrate, 0 g fat, 0 g saturated fat, 2 g fiber, 27 g sugar*

CLASSIC MSC REJUVENATION SHAKE

- 8 ounces mineral water (noncarbonated)
- 5 ice cubes
- ½ cup mixed fresh berries, frozen
- 1 scoop vanilla Designer Protein powder

In a blender, combine the water, ice cubes, berries, and protein powder. Blend on high speed for 45 seconds. Serve immediately. *Makes 1 serving. Per serving: 232 calories, 17 g protein, 38 g carbohydrate, 1 g fat, 0 g saturated fat, 3 g fiber, 28 g sugar*

VARIATION

Chocolate-Berry Delight: Use chocolate protein powder in place of vanilla.

MSC POWER ENERGY BOOST

- 6 ounces very strong coffee
- 2 ounces fat-free milk
- 5 ice cubes
- 1 scoop Designer Protein powder (chocolate or vanilla)

In a blender, combine the coffee, milk, ice cubes, and protein powder. Blend on high speed for 45 seconds. Serve immediately. *Makes 1 serving. Per serving: 143 calories, 20 g protein, 12 g carbohydrate, 2 g fat, 0 g saturated fat, 1 g fiber, 3 g sugar*

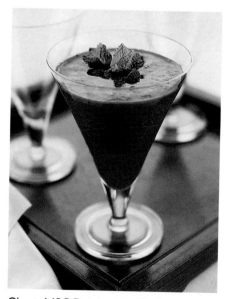

Classic MSC Rejuvenation Shake

A SOUND EATING PLAN

Now you have the tools you need to make the best eating choices in any situation. Learning the correct food choices to make will take you far along your path to a Sound Mind and Body. As you venture down your path to wellness, remember to take small steps. This is a life change, not a quick fix.

On the following pages, you'll find 2 weeks' worth of meal plans incorporating the recipes I've given you. These plans give you about 1,200 calories a day. You should drink at least 8 ounces of water with each of your meals (plus enough in between to equal 64 ounces per day); remember that adding drinks such as sports drinks and fruit juice will add calories and slow your progress.

Day 1

Breakfast
Asparagus Frittata

Turkey sausage (2 links)

Chocolate-Berry Delight Protein Shake

Lunch
2 ounces fresh turkey breast with 1 slice Oven-Dried Tomato

½ cup Chickpea Salad with Salsa Fresca on 1 cup raw spinach with 1 tablespoon Lemon Burst Vinaigrette

Snack
4 ounces chicken breast

1 apple

Dinner
Almond-Crusted Catfish

Quinoa Salad with 2 tablespoons Ginger Soy Dressing

Citrus-Mint Salad

Day 2

Breakfast
2 cups Kellogg's All-Bran Extra Fiber bran flakes with 8 ounces fat-free milk

8 ounces yogurt with ¼ cup fresh berries

Lunch
Chicken Papaya Salad

Black Bean–Roasted Red Pepper Soup

Snack
½ cup broccoli dipped in ¼ cup Fat-Free Ranch Dressing

Dinner
Turkey Meat Loaf

Cauliflower Hash

1 cup steamed spinach

Sunburst Baked Apple with Cinnamon Stick

Day 3

Breakfast

1½ cups plain oatmeal

Turkey sausage (2 links)

Lunch

Tuna Salad Niçoise

2 tablespoons Citrus Cilantro Dressing

¾ cup No-Fat Hummus

Snack

8 ounces yogurt with ¼ cup fresh berries

1 ounce almonds

Dinner

Roasted Chilean Sea Bass with Vidalia
    Onions and Summer Squash

Couscous Salad

Green Melon and Parsley Granita

Day 4

Breakfast

MSC Breakfast Wrap

David's Plain and Simple Protein Shake

Lunch

½ cup lentil beans over 2 cups spinach

2 tablespoons Herb Balsamic Vinaigrette

1 ounce almonds

Snack

1 fresh peach

Dinner

Shiitake Chicken Paillard

Roasted Vegetable Caponata

Citrus-Mint Salad

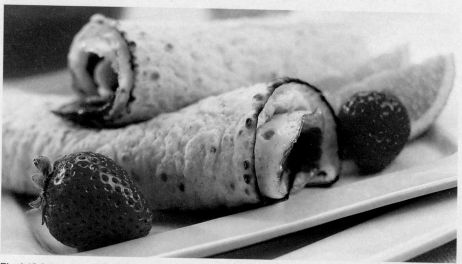

The MSC Breakfast Wrap (p. 168)

Day 5

Breakfast

Classic MSC Rejuvenation Shake

2 hard-boiled eggs

Lunch

Thai Ginger Sirloin Salad

Snack

8 ounces yogurt with ¼ cup fresh berries

1 ounce almonds

Dinner

Cod Cakes

No-Fat Hummus

Poached Pears

Day 6

Breakfast

Classic Egg-White Omelette

Turkey bacon (2 slices)

MSC Power Energy Boost

Lunch

Honeydew Tomatillo Soup

¾ cup fresh veggies (cauliflower,
    broccoli, green peppers) dipped in
    ¼ cup Spicy Peanut Sauce

Snack

1 ounce sunflower seeds

2 ounces tuna with 1 teaspoon Dijon
    mustard

Dinner

Turkey Meatballs with Spaghetti Squash
    Marinara

1 cup steamed kale

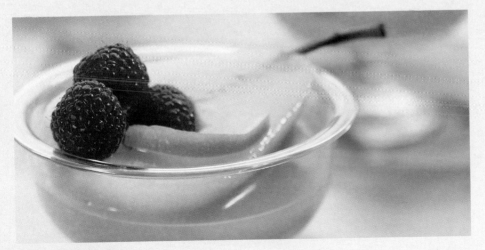

Poached Pears (p. 192)

Day 7

Breakfast

2 cups Kellogg's All-Bran Extra Fiber
    bran flakes with 8 ounces fat-free milk

8 ounces yogurt with ¼ cup fresh berries

Lunch

Chickpea Salad with Salsa Fresca

2 cups Romaine lettuce

Snack

1 apple

Turkey bacon (2 slices)

Dinner

Seared Tuna with Spicy Wasabi Slaw

1 cup steamed kale

Day 8

Breakfast

MSC Breakfast Wrap

8 ounces yogurt with ¼ cup fresh berries

Lunch

Gazpacho with 2 grilled shrimp

½ cup lentil beans over 2 cups spinach

2 tablespoons Herb Balsamic Vinegar

Snack

Preworkout Fruit Shake

½ ounce pumpkin seeds

Dinner

Sesame Salmon

Tomato Shallot Salad

1 cup steamed collard greens

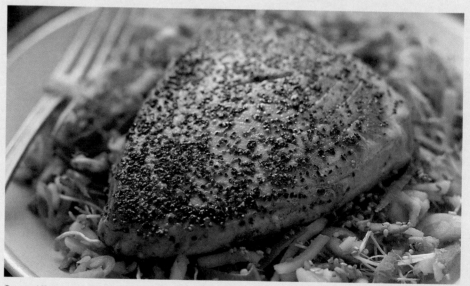

Seared Tuna with Spicy Wasabi Slaw (p. 187)

Day 9

Breakfast

Huevos Rancheros

Turkey sausage (2 links)

Lunch

2 ounces poached salmon mixed with 2 tablespoons fat-free yogurt and ¼ cup chopped roasted peppers

2 cups mixed greens

2 tablespoons Strawberry Vinaigrette

1 ounce toasted sesame seeds

10 reduced-fat tortilla chips

Snack

¾ cup fresh veggies dipped in Summer Salsa

David's Plain and Simple Protein Shake

Dinner

Herb-Crusted Turkey Breast

Cauliflower Mushroom Mash

1 cup steamed spinach

Sunburst Baked Apple with Cinnamon Stick

Day 10

Breakfast

MSC Power Energy Boost

Classic Egg-White Omelette made with ½ cup broccoli and ¼ cup fat-free Cheddar cheese

Lunch

Roasted Turkey Basil Salad

¼ cup each brown rice and black beans

Snack

1 orange

1 ounce almonds

Dinner

Halibut Niçoise

2 cups mesclun greens

½ cup haricot verts

3 tablespoons Balsamic Vinaigrette

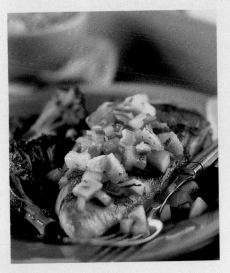

Summer Salsa (p. 170) and Asian Broccoli Stir-Fry (p. 191).

Day 11

Breakfast

Asparagus Frittata

Turkey sausage (2 links)

MSC Power Energy Boost

Lunch

½ cup quinoa over 2 cups mesclun greens

2 tablespoons Ginger Soy Dressing

6 ounces tuna

Snack

½ cup cottage cheese (2%)

Dinner

Chicken Satay

Cucumber Salad

Strawberry-Raspberry Granita

Day 12

Breakfast

2 cups Kellogg's All-Bran Extra Fiber
   bran flakes with 8 ounces fat-free milk

2 scrambled egg whites

1 ounce reduced-fat Cheddar cheese

Lunch

Spicy Thai Shrimp Salad

1 cup steamed asparagus

1 pear

Snack

1 cup chopped fresh vegetables
   (cucumbers, cauliflower, cherry
   tomatoes) dipped in ½ cup Fat-Free
   Ranch Dressing

8 ounces yogurt with ¼ cup fresh berries

1 ounce almonds

Dinner

Grilled Tuna with Arugula and Vidalia
   Onions

½ cup brown rice with ½ cup mushrooms

Asian Broccoli Stir-Fry

¼ cup fresh berries

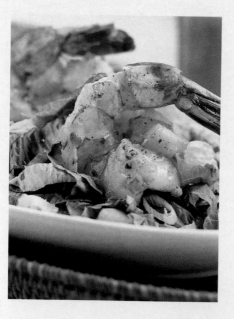

Spicy Thai Shrimp Salad (p. 175)

Day 13

Breakfast

Huevos Rancheros

8 ounces yogurt with ¼ cup fresh berries

Lunch

Black Bean–Roasted Red Pepper Soup

4 ounces grilled chicken

1 orange

Snack

1 ounce tofu

½ cup spinach with 1 tablespoon Lemon
    Burst Vinaigrette

Dinner

Turkey Chili

Roasted Brussel Sprouts

½ cup pureed edamame

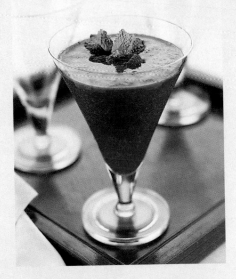

Day 14

Breakfast

Classic Egg-White Omelette

Turkey bacon (2 slices)

1 ounce reduced-fat Cheddar cheese

Lunch

Chicken salad made with 2 ounces
    poached chicken breast,
    2 tablespoons Dijon mustard,
    1 tablespoon nonfat plain yogurt,
    1 tablespoon Madison Square Club
    Herb Blend, ¼ cup diced celery,
    ¼ cup chopped bell pepper

Mixed greens

Black Bean–Roasted Red Pepper Soup

Snack

Classic MSC Rejuvenation Shake

1 ounce almonds

Dinner

Broiled trout with Fat-Free Horseradish
    Cream Sauce

1 cup steamed broccoli rabe

Green Melon and Parsley Granita

Classic MSC Rejuvenation Shake (p. 194)

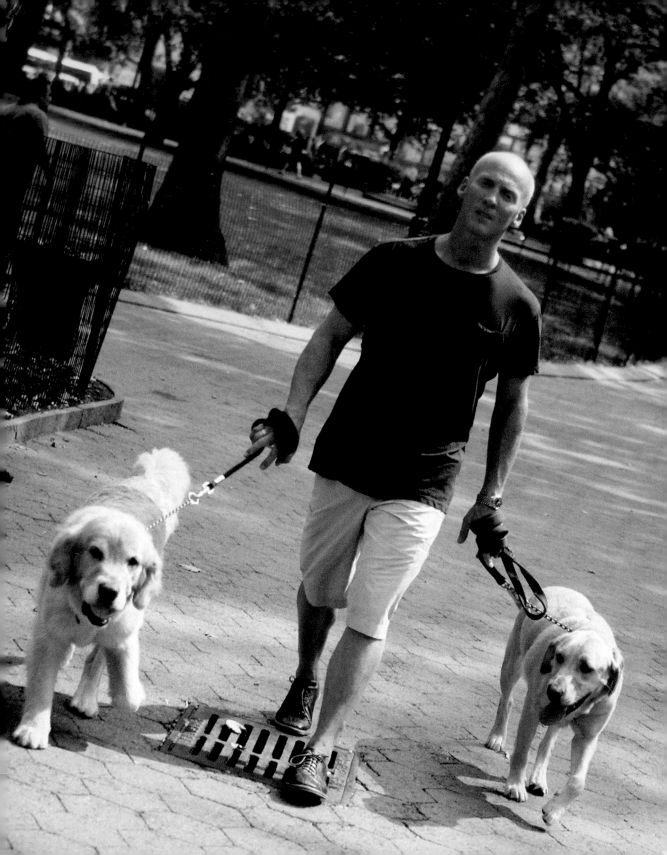

Chapter Five

SOUND THINKING

AFTER one of my clients had lost more than 100 pounds, her true battle began. "I've been in this place before," she told me. "I've lost weight before, and because of that, I know that losing it is only a small part of the battle. The difficulty is keeping it off and not sabotaging all the work that I've done."

About a week later, she stood me up for her training session. She didn't even call to cancel. Like many people, her inner demons were sabotaging her fitness and eating habits.

I knew she needed to start a Sound Thinking training program. So I called her, spent an hour with her on the phone, promised to help her deal with her emotional eating, and got her back on her training schedule the following week.

On your path to wellness, what goes on inside your head is just as important as the food you eat and the exercises you complete. To maintain the results you get with my Sound Eating and Sound Training programs, you must make a deep internal change that will flip your motivation switch, helping you stay on your wellness program for the rest of your life. That change involves Sound Thinking.

For example, do your emotions affect your eating? Do you eat when you are angry, sad, frustrated, or stressed? Or do you get so stressed at work that you have no energy to work out after work? Are you sometimes so depressed that you can't motivate yourself to get off the couch? If you don't address the reasons you eat the way you do or the way you live your life, you won't be able to maintain your results.

These inner demons never really go away. Much like fat cells, they shrink until you no longer notice them. But they are still there, waiting to find a weakness in your new Sound Mind, Body, and Spirit. The stronger you are physically and mentally, the tougher it will be for those demons to break through. I believe so strongly in my Sound Mind philosophy that many of my clients call me their Zen trainer. To help you stay on track long-term, I offer you the six keys to Sound Thinking, which you can incorporate into your own lifestyle over the next 6 weeks.

WEEK 1: INNER PRESENCE

When one of my clients decided that she was going to lose weight and get fit, she signed herself up for a 3-week spa vacation where she planned to exercise, eat healthy foods, and lose weight. The vacation was a month-and-a-half away. Each day, she would wake up, look in the mirror, and feel disgusted about herself. And she waited for that spa vacation to fix it all.

Finally, one day she asked herself, "What am I waiting for?" She read about my club, made a phone call, and signed up for a training session the following day. By the time her spa

vacation rolled around, she was in the best shape of her life.

Like her, many people live in the future. Clients often tell me, "I'm going to start exercising next week" and "I'll make smarter food choices tomorrow" and "Next time I won't be so angry." And it goes on and on.

I often respond: "Time travel hasn't been invented yet. If you want to live a Sound life, stay out of the future and concentrate on the present moment."

I learned about Inner Presence the hard way back in the early 1990s when my best friend, my uncle, and my aunt all died of sudden illnesses over the course of 2 years. Those deaths shook me hard, forcing me to face my own mortality. I realized that none of us are guaranteed to live another hour, day, week, month, or year. Yet, we often take that time for granted. I stopped taking time for granted and began seeing it as a precious gift that could run out at any second. I began living in the moment.

Living in the present moment has its roots in both Eastern and Western religions. The renowned Vietnamese Buddhist monk Thich Nhat Hanh once wrote the following mantra: "Waking up this morning, I smile. Twenty-four brand-new hours are before me. I vow to live fully in each moment and to look at all beings with eyes of compassion."

A well-known story from Western religion is that of God revealing himself to Moses at the burning bush. In the Bible, God tells Moses that his name is "I AM," not "I WAS" or "I WILL BE." In other words, when you live in the present, you will always have the safety and comfort of God, but when you live in the future or the past, you will struggle.

Living in the present does more than bring you peace of mind. It helps you concentrate on what is most important to you, such as your fitness and eating goals. But how do you get there? How do you stop worrying about the future and regretting the past? Life consists of a series of choices. To live in the present moment, we must prioritize those choices. Using your notebook to record your answers, try these exercises to get started.

Inner Presence Exercise #1

Stop procrastinating. Make a list of all of the things you want to accomplish by the time you die. Put a deadline on each goal.

Inner Presence Exercise #2

Think about how you would feel if your doctor told you that you had just 1 day to live. How would you feel about those unfinished goals?

Inner Presence Exercise #3

In the space below, write how you want to be remembered after you die. Then assess your life so far and think about what you have done to create that legacy. How are you doing? How do you need to change your life and life choices?

Inner Presence Exercise #4

This week, every time you find yourself putting off something important on your legacy list, think about how you might act differently if you knew you were going to die tomorrow. At the end of my days, whether I'm 40 or 50 or 80, I want to know that I made a difference, that I pushed myself to the limit. I want to feel proud of my accomplishments, and I want the people I've left behind to feel the same.

WEEK 2: INNER STRENGTH

Martial artists often talk about inner strength. Without calling upon it, they would not be able to muster the physical strength to break a board with a single punch. They would not be able to defeat an opponent with a single stare. They definitely would not be able to resist that pepperoni pizza or hot fudge sundae.

Some martial artists say that when they take that inner strength to its highest level, they can project it into any situation, such as scaring an aggressive dog into submission, emerging as a natural leader in business, or commanding respect from each and every person they meet.

Attaining this inner strength doesn't take years of study in martial arts or a black belt in karate. You can build and harness this same inner strength in your workouts, at your job, with your friends, and in your relationships.

What exactly is inner strength? It's an inner can-do attitude. It's the belief that you can do anything you set your mind to. Simply put, what you believe influences what you will accomplish. Before a martial artist punches a board, he sees himself breaking it. He knows he will break it. Then he breaks it. His visualization, confidence, and strength combine to break the board.

This is the same confidence that you need to maintain your new wellness program. Study after study shows that self-efficacy—the belief that you can stick with it—is one of the most important determining factors in whether someone maintains a new habit. That same inner can-do attitude will also help you finish that last pushup, complete your first full pullup, or run an extra 10 minutes on the treadmill.

Not convinced? Then think about this notable experiment. Researchers picked a number of students at random and told their teachers that the students possessed genetic traits that would allow them to excel academically. In reality, the students were not any smarter than the others in the class. But by the end of the year, they had excelled academically because their teachers believed in them, passing on that confidence to the students themselves.

The power of inner strength also can affect your health. Many studies show that confidence or optimism is one of the most important deciding factors in whether you suffer a stroke or heart attack. People who believe in themselves and their abilities live longer than those who don't.

Simply put, if you will it, it can be done. So how do you learn to trust your own abilities? How do you harness your inner strength? Try the following exercises.

Inner Strength Exercise #1

Surround yourself with positive messages. I grew up with parents who told me that I could accomplish anything I set my mind to. I lived in a world where "can't" wasn't in the dictionary. Think of the people you associate with daily. Who encourages you to be your best, and who holds you back? As you build your inner strength, gravitate to the former. The world is full of negative energy. Surrounding yourself with positive friends and acquaintances will help you to counter the negativity that you can't control.

Inner Strength Exercise #2

On the day I went to take the bar exam, I listened to a tape with positive, confidence-building songs such as "Believe in Yourself" from *The Wiz*. It may seem a little silly, but the more positive your surroundings, the more confident you'll feel about your abilities. Make a tape of inspiring songs and listen to it often, especially when you feel a bout of "I can'ts" coming on. If music isn't your thing, try reading poetry or Bible verses.

Inner Strength Exercise #3

I learned to trust my own inner strength when I was studying for the bar exam after law school. Lots of people unconsciously tried to fill my head with negative thoughts—reminding me that 35 percent of those who take the exam fail on their first try. But I was determined. I spent 7 weeks straight studying for that exam. And I passed the bar on my first try.

I look back at that experience and realize that law school was a series of tests for me. It took me years to realize that I needed to take and pass those tests in order to move on to the next level in my growth process. We all need challenges, and part of our growth centers on finding those challenges and meeting them head on.

In your notebook, list all of your major accomplishments. Write down everything that took willpower and focus to complete, from making the cheerleading squad or football team in high school to landing your first job. Then list all of the hard times you have survived, from the death of a loved one to a long illness to the loss of a job. If you survived that, just think what else you can do.

You must not forget that out of every negative experience you can glean some positive energy. You must step back and examine the situation in order to fully grasp what is going on. It is only through this analytical approach that you will be able to bear the situations that seem to be the most unbearable.

Inner Strength Exercise #4

Any time this week when you catch yourself thinking "I can't," replace that thought with "I can if I break it down into doable steps." Then take out your notebook, write down the steps you'll need to take, and start taking them. For example, you might not be strong enough to do a full pushup. So start by doing it on your knees, then doing it against a wall, and then doing it on the balls of your feet.

Inner Strength Exercise #5

Look for encouragement from high places. When I opened my test for the bar exam, the first essay question was one that I had worked on during a study class. Some people might call this a simple coincidence, but I call it a God-incidence. And I took it as a sign from above that I was going to pass the test.

I've always felt that I have a guardian angel watching over me. Keep your eyes and heart open for your "angel's" voice. As you listen, your angel will make its presence felt. For example, when I watched the birth of my niece (and goddaughter)

Samantha, I felt that something about her was magical. She came into this world a few years after the deaths of my aunt, uncle, and best friend. After a few dark years, her birth pulled me out of the doldrums. I held her when she was just 1 minute old. Samantha represented all that was good and pure and innocent in life. She made it all make sense. She stared in my eyes with such intensity that I suddenly realized that life was about living.

In your notebook, list some of your God-incidences.

Inner Strength Exercise #6

Too often, people see failure as something that destroys their inner strength. But I want you to look at failure as a way to learn more about yourself. Anytime something doesn't go as planned or you feel that you didn't accomplish a goal, ask yourself:

1. Did I do the best I could to my ability in this situation? If the answer is yes, then you didn't fail. If you've done your best, you can't ask for more from yourself. But if you haven't done your best, proceed to question 2.

2. What could I have done differently to succeed in that situation? Every situation, if viewed in a positive light, is there to teach you something. There is no purely negative situation, just your perception of a negative situation. For example, if you fail to stay

on my meal plan, you may feel as if you've done something negative or bad. But you can convert that to a positive by understanding the reasons for the breakdown and getting back on the plan. Every positive response to a potential breakdown makes you stronger. Remember, as my mom always said, "What doesn't kill you makes you stronger."

WEEK 3: INNER ENERGY

According to the Eastern religion of Tao, tortoises possess an amazing ability: They are incredibly efficient energy nurturers. The ability to create and store this energy has allowed tortoises to live for 100 years or more on very little food, the Taoists say.

Tortoises nurture energy by making smart use of their shells. A tortoise will draw into its shell to rest, hide from danger, and generate energy. Even though we humans don't have a visible shell, we can still create energy by drawing into ourselves.

Every interaction in life requires an exchange of energy. In some interactions, you receive energy. In others, you give it away. Sometimes it's good to give away energy, such as when you're comforting a friend in need. Sometimes you give away energy wastefully, such as when you get steamed at a coworker or fight with your spouse. In those situations, you would do much better to first create an energy reserve, and like the tortoise, draw into your protective shell.

Too often, we behave as if we have no shell or barrier against the outer world. We don't take a step back to shrink into our shell and think; we simply react and give away energy that we might not have to give. Act, don't react. I like to think that I spend my life acting and not reacting to the things and people around me. By doing this, I reserve and conserve my energy and use it in the most efficient way.

How can you act more like the tortoise and conserve your energy? Try this exercise.

Inner Energy Exercise

This week, pay attention to the times you feel your heart racing, your face flushing, your palms sweating, and your anger or frustration brewing. Before you react, shrink into your shell. While in your protective shell:

1. Take a few deep breaths. Deep breathing promotes clear thinking.

2. Ask yourself, "What is this interaction about? Why do I feel this way? What is the best way for me to respond? Where are my priorities at this moment?"

3. If you're feeling so overwhelmed that no immediate answers come to you, take out a sheet of paper and write down all the things that are making you feel overwhelmed. Then look at each item and carefully decide which needs to be tackled right now and which can wait until later. Re-

Meditation and You

Meditation is the perfect way to step back from the world into a protective shell. Meditating regularly will open you to your physical inner self, helping you develop a Sound Mind.

Some meditation gurus will tell you to clear your mind of all extraneous thoughts, that the quieter your mind, the more expert you are at meditating. Others tell you to zero in on your breath, your heartbeat, or a sound in the room. Others have you visualize a white light. Still others have you think about relaxing each muscle in your body.

Which guru is right? They all are. There is no one right way to meditate, as long as how you meditate brings you a sense of restful calm. I like to go to a beautiful place, listen to music through headphones, and let my mind wander. That's what works for me. Some people meditate at the top of mountains. Others do it during a ride in the subway. Meditation is individual to the individual in you.

member: You won't always get every-thing done on your to-do list. That's normal.

If you first take a step back and allow yourself to think, you'll react in a much more positive manner, which will result in a more positive out-come. The thinking is the part that's often overlooked, and it's the part that allows you to maintain your en-ergy rather than waste it.

WEEK 4: INNER MEANING

When my mother used the adage "What doesn't kill you makes you stronger," she meant that every nega-tive situation in life can be turned into a positive, helping you accom-plish greater things later in life.

You find strength in tragedy by searching for the meaning of it all. I've always been a spiritual person, and I've always believed in God. So I often ask God, "What do you want from me? Why are you doing this?" And then suddenly it makes sense.

In the early 1990s, after losing my aunt, my uncle, and my best friend, I felt as if God was sending me a mes-sage along with all of the tragedy around me. The message was that life is short and I had better start living it to my fullest potential. That's when I started incorporating spiritual well-ness into my training programs.

I actually emerged from this period of personal tragedy with a stronger resolve and raison d'être. These three people all meant so much to me. I loved them all very much, and their losses at first seemed painful and sense-less. With time, however, their deaths made me even more determined to love every moment to the fullest and surround myself with positive people who give off positive energy. I wasn't going to waste one moment of my life. Living life to the fullest potential be-came my mission. It became my Inner Meaning. And it's one of the reasons I decided to write this book.

How can you find meaning in hardship? Try this exercise.

Inner Meaning Exercise

Writing down your answers to the following questions in your notebook will help you find the inner meaning in tough situations.

What is your hardship?

How do you feel?

What could you learn from this sit-uation? Is there a lesson in it from God?

WEEK 5: INNER PASSION

I didn't always know what I wanted to be when I grew up, and I spent many of my adult years trying to figure that out. I drifted from working odd jobs to considering running my own catering business to becoming a lawyer. But none of those careers made me happy. None of them made me feel fulfilled. None of them were right for me. It wasn't until I began training people that I discovered my inner passion for nurturing others. Throughout my life I have been a nurturing person. Even as a small child I changed my baby sister's diaper in the middle of the night so her cries wouldn't wake my parents. Nurturing others is my passion. It's my life's purpose, and it fits right in with what I do on the training floor.

Many people live most of their lives as if they were robots, going through the motions at work and in their relationships. They feel little inner passion. It's not that the passion isn't there; they are just not tapping it. If only they tapped that passion, their lives would become so much more fulfilling.

People often fear passion. It is misunderstood and sometimes applied in the wrong way toward the wrong things. But the clearer your path and the stronger your passion, the greater your chances of success.

Inner passion makes life much more clear, easy, and meaningful. When you live your passion, everything falls into place, and it opens up energy for you to pursue your wellness goals of eating healthy and exercising. We all have to find our passion, strive for the best, and most important, live a fulfilled life that exudes goodness and spirituality. We are

---

Sound Mind, Sound Body Success Story

Before I started training with David, I spent 3 years exercising very little and eating poorly. I was overweight, felt tired all the time, and was sometimes at odds with my colleagues and family. Now, I've lost weight and firmed up. But most important, I've changed the way I live my life. While working with David, I began to understand that happiness is based on following your life's calling.

As CEO of a major company, I was consumed with trying to be the best CEO I could be. But then I realized that what truly makes me happy is the deal-making aspects of buying and selling companies. So I refocused what I do at the company so that I could become more involved in making deals.

Now, when I wake up in the morning, I feel at one with who I am. I'm doing what truly makes me happy, and I have more energy, focus, and balance because of it.

—Todd Hamilton

all born with amazing possibilities. What are yours? Try the following exercises.

Inner Passion Exercise #1

You can discover your inner passion by answering the following questions in your notebook:

1. Think back to your childhood. What came naturally to you as a child? What traits did people see in you?

2. What traits do you continue to see in yourself today?

3. When do you feel happiest and content? What needs are you satisfying?

4. How can you rearrange your life to bring out your natural, God-given passion?

Once you discover your inner passion and start changing your life accordingly, I challenge you to live your life with integrity. At the end of each day, spend a few moments of quiet reflection and think about what you did that day and how it relates to your strength of character and passion. Did you follow your passion today?

Inner Passion Exercise #2

Many people are driven not by passion but by other, less invigorating pursuits. At one point in my life, I was driven by success, recognition, and even money. That's why I studied so hard to become a lawyer. But those drives didn't satisfy my inner needs, and ultimately that's why I left the field of law to become a Wellness Trainer.

I like to call these things empty drives. None of them come from your core, and none of them satisfy your soul. Here's a list of empty drives. Check off how many apply to you, and then think about how they have affected your choices in life and how they interfere with your inner passion.

☐ Pleasing others

☐ Recognition

☐ Making money

☐ Spending money

☐ Owning things

☐ Wielding power

WEEK 6: INNER PEACE

Once I realized the precious nature of time, I also decided that life was too short to waste on negativity. True, every once in a while I have a bad day and feel down because of it. But rarely do I ever allow myself to stay down for long. It's a waste of time, and I'm in better health because of it.

Negative emotions—anger, sadness, jealousy, depression, frustration, worry, anxiety . . . you name it—all drain your energy, and they all put you at a higher risk for disease. Some things are worth feeling sad about, but many are not. If you're still brewing over the short shrift you felt the doorman gave you this morning, you need to get your inner peace in order.

So how do you change your emotions? By slowing down, noticing them, and taking corrective action. The Chinese have a phrase, *pu shih*, which means that you accept what comes in life, whether you perceive it to be positive or negative. You create negative emotions when you fight this acceptance. To develop your inner peace, try the following exercises.

Inner Peace Exercise #1

Keep an emotion journal for the week. Pay particular attention to your negative, energy-draining emotions, such as anger, frustration, depression, and jealousy. Write down the circumstances surrounding your emotions.

At the end of the week, read your journal. Were any of the circumstances truly worthy of wallowing in negativity? If not, how else might you have responded?

Inner Peace Exercise #2

Whenever you catch yourself thinking negatively, perform an act of love. You can start with people whom you find easy to love. For example, you might try calling your grandmother just to say hello. But progress to doing an act of love for the person who was instrumental in bringing on your negative thinking, whether it's your boss, a coworker, your spouse, or a service person. For example, if you're receiving abysmal service at a restaurant, instead of berating the waitress, try being the little pearl in her day. You'll be amazed at how changing your response can make all the difference in your temperament.

THE NEXT STEP

You are almost finished with your wellness journey. It is my hope that after reading this chapter, you will feel as I do: Anything is possible. All you need to do when you meet a barrier—any barrier—is examine it, break it down, and deal with it one step at a time. And remember, when you feel particularly overwhelmed, I am only as far away as this book.

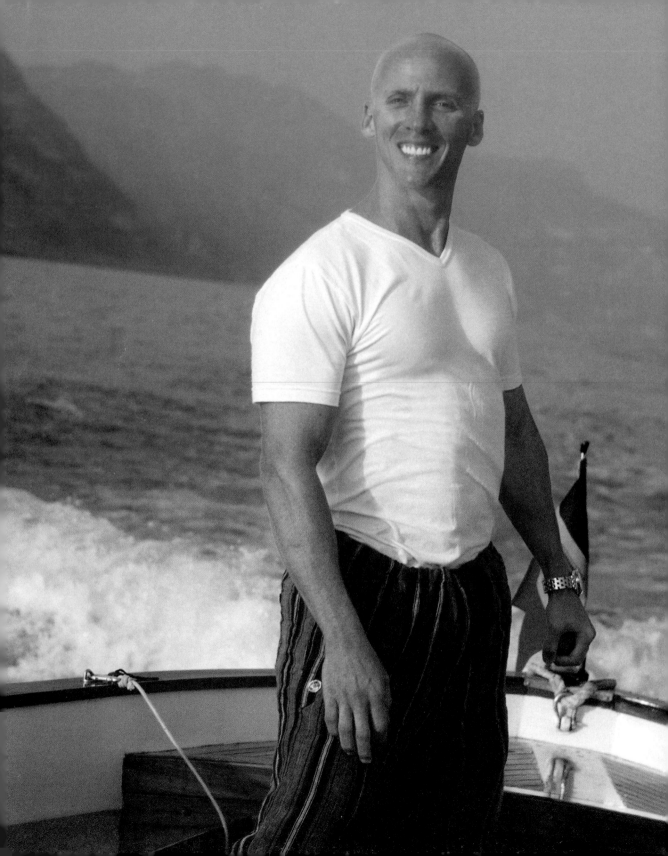

Chapter Six

SOUND LIVING

YOU'VE SUCCESSFULLY traversed the first five steps of my Sound Mind, Sound Body program, and you've transformed your exercise, eating, and thinking habits. You should feel extremely pleased with yourself for getting this far. Your new Sound habits are creating a fitter, firmer, sexier you. Congratulations!

You may have already navigated some rough spots in your journey. But the roughest section is still to come. You see, the first 6 weeks of any new program are usually the easiest. That's when your resolve is strongest, your results are most dramatic, and your positive reinforcement from friends and family is highest. It's beyond the 6 weeks where your true endurance test begins.

Research shows that most people quit their wellness habits not during the first 6 weeks or even the first 6

months—what they call the adoption phase—but during the maintenance, or what I call the rest-of-your life phase.

It takes true commitment and resolve to navigate the rest-of-your-life phase of your Sound Mind, Sound Body program. Yet that commitment and that resolve will feel a bit easier if you first plan for the most common barriers to your success.

According to research, the most common reasons people quit new wellness programs during the maintenance phase include a change of work responsibilities or hours, vacations, sudden changes in health, and strained relationships with family and friends. This final step in your Sound Mind, Sound Body program will help you traverse such rough patches as if they were paved road, keeping you firmly aligned with your path to success.

To finish building your Sound foundation, you need to take step six in your Sound Mind, Sound Body program. For this step, you'll find ways to expand your Sound teachings beyond your home gym and kitchen. You'll infuse your entire life with Soundness, helping you to make Sound decisions in every aspect of your life, from the vacations you take to the parties you throw to the food you store in your desk drawer. In all, you'll be better equipped to fight your self-sabotaging inner demons.

LIVING SOUNDLY AT WORK

As a high-tech executive, Michelle Blank frequently works 12-hour days. And some days are more stressful than others. During the afternoon of a particularly stressful day, Michelle needed a break. She went to the corner store and bought not one, not two, not three, but *four* candy bars, and she ate them. All.

But she got back on track. "For an entire year, I had not done anything like that. But what was amazing was that I ate those four candy bars, and the next day, I was right back at the gym and following my healthy eating habits again," she said. "Had that happened to me before I started this program, I would have felt like, 'I've just eaten four candy bars. What's the point?' And my program would have been over."

That's why work stress poses the biggest roadblock along your path to

success. Not only does it encourage you to slack off on your fitness program— "because I don't have time"—and to eat cruddy foods—"because they make me feel better"—but it also fries your brain, preventing you from realizing that a little slipup is just that—a slipup.

Stress weakens your lock on that inner demon who is always struggling to get out. The stronger you are, the clearer you are. The more you realize that, the more invincible you will become. While spending long hours writing this book and simultaneously running my training business and developing a full line of spa products, I have come face-to-face with my own inner demon, who definitely knows which buttons to push. But as my friend and client Chris, a prominent psychiatrist, tells me, "Most people never expose their inner demons, and go through life in a state of bewilderment. It is through the process of first exposing them and then defeating them that you will find true strength and wellness."

For all of us, the battle is lifelong but definitely surmountable.

During the rest of your Sound life, you will slip up. We all do. From time to time, I even slip on my own wellness program. As a chronic overachiever, I tend to take on too much. I routinely get by on too little sleep, and consequently, each morning I set out with the same goal: to complete the day with inner tranquillity. But sometimes, busyness prevails and I get off track. I'll allow stress, the ringing phone, and demanding clients to throw me off my routine. In order to call people back or address their concerns, I'll eat up some of my personal time. And then I'll get mad at myself for doing so.

One night 2 weeks before my deadline for this book, I was overcome with fear and panic. What was I doing writing a book? Would anyone read this? Fear is often paralyzing but not necessarily bad. A dear friend and mentor, Ralph, told me just days before I opened my club: "Without fear, one never succeeds." We all have some self-doubt, especially when dealing with our careers and livelihoods. The key is in how we deal with it.

Along the road to spiritual wellness, it is the process of accepting self-doubt and our limitations and striving forward that makes the difference. My life's lessons have taught me that even the most seemingly impossible situations and tasks can be made tolerable if approached logically. So whenever I'm feeling overwhelmed or scared or tense, I take a deep breath, realize my error of judgment, and get myself back on track.

There will be times that you will blow off your fitness for the day or week or month. You will eat too much of something—and wish later that you hadn't. When that happens, just move on. Remember: Live in the moment, not in the past. You may never be able to totally eliminate stress-induced slipups, but you certainly can prevent many of them.

Count to three. Anytime you feel frenzied at work and find yourself craving a candy bar, try this three-step technique:

1. Stop what you are doing.

2. Take three slow, deep breaths. Nothing else restores lucid thinking faster than awareness of your breath. Breath is one of the most calming mechanisms you have at your disposal. Simply switching to deep breathing for a few seconds can help you weather almost any storm. I recommend even taking a few minutes before your workout to take some deep, cleansing breaths to get rid of the tension of the day.

3. Focus on the positive. I like the saying by Eleanor Roosevelt that no one can make you feel inferior without your consent. Try to find the smallest bit of positive from any negative. For example, if you can't get a project done on time, remember that next time, you'll have learned to do the work faster. Turning negatives into positives is a difficult mental challenge, but not an impossible one. Soon the anger, frustration, or stress will be out of your system, and you'll be ready to face the day with renewed Soundness. Just like lifting a heavier weight makes your muscles stronger, the process of gleaning positive from the negative makes you spiritually and mentally stronger.

Work out where you are. If you're the type of person who works 15-hour days or spends every other night in a hotel, you will need a flexible fitness plan. My Sound Training and Eating programs can be done anytime, anywhere—whether you are traveling on business or stuck working late at the office. Just modify your program to meet your individual needs. Here are some ways to stay fit on the road or in the office:

1. Use your weight. My training program offers numerous body-weight exercises, many designed specifically by me, that you can do in any hotel room. Pushups are the quintessential body-weight exercise, but you can also stay fit with the crab, the platypus walk, scissors, dips, sumo lunges, jump squats, the reverse crab, and more.

2. Use whatever weight you can find. For traditional moves, you can use some items in your hotel room or office to your advantage. Try pressing the desk chair, for example.

3. Pack some weight. You don't want to lug your entire set of dumbbells around, but what about a set of ankle weights? Store a pair in your office and pack a pair in your suitcase. You can wrap your ankle weights around your wrists or hold them in your hands to offer more resistance for side and front raises, for example.

4. Take it outside. For your aerobic fitness, try walking or jogging through the parking lot, running the stairwells, or even jogging up and down the hallways of your office building or hotel.

Pack a good desk. If you're stuck at work for 12 or more hours, you're going to need quality food on hand. Fill your desk with healthy nonperish-

---

Workday Workout

Whether you're stuck working long hours in a cubicle or stranded at an airport hotel, the following workout will keep you fit:

1. Squats
2. Lunges
3. Side Lunges
4. Scissors
5. David's Donkey Deluxe or David's Deluxe Floor Routine

6. Incline Pushups on your desk
7. Dips on your desk
8. Side and Front Raises using ankle weights
9. Biceps Curls using wrist weights
10. Crunches
11. Good Mornings

The 5-Minute Workout

Everyone has bad days when no matter what, you simply can't find 30 to 45 minutes to work out. On those days, take 5. You can keep your muscles toned and strong by doing as many Pushups, Knee Bends (Squats without weight), and Crunches as you can fit into 5 minutes.

ables such as protein bars, apples, nuts, protein shake powder, and so on. If you have access to a refrigerator or freezer, spend 1 day each weekend making up a number of personal healthy frozen dinners. Each Sunday, cook up a storm and store the goods in airtight containers, then eat them throughout the week. You can also store milk, yogurt, and berries in the fridge to use for shakes. I like to keep a box of brown rice on hand at all times. And I like to roast two or three sweet potatoes at a time and then store them in the fridge at work to be eaten in case of an emergency. Whatever you do, stay away from chips, raisins, jelly beans, granola bars, and other snack foods that are either mostly fat or mostly sugar.

YOUR FITNESS VACATION

When people go on vacation, they tend to leave their Sound lifestyles behind and embark on weeklong eating and sleeping binges. Something about the word "vacation" creates an I-can-eat-anything-I-want-and-stop-exercising-if-I-feel-like-it attitude for most people.

There are long afternoons in lounge chairs nibbling cheese and crackers, and huge restaurant meals complete with fatty appetizers, carbo-hydrate-dense main dishes, and deca-dent desserts. The beer and wine make an appearance earlier and earlier each day. And the caffeine gets stronger and stronger each morning.

Most people return home de-pressed, worn out, and chubby. None of their clothes fit.

Have I just described every vaca-tion you've ever taken? Don't feel bad; I've taken the same gluttonous vacations. So have all of my clients.

Not too long ago, I tried a different approach to vacations. I gathered some friends and clients and took them on a 10-day luxury trip to Greece. We trav-eled aboard an 85-foot private yacht with a crew and a chef who prepared the most healthy and delicious foods with a local, Turkish flair.

We started in the town of Mar-maris, sailed along the Turkish coast, and mountain climbed, swam, and ran during each trip ashore. We started

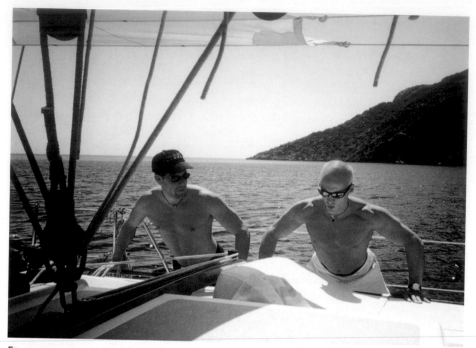

Fitness at sea

each morning with a brisk swim or run, followed by protein shakes and herbs and vitamins. Though each day was slightly different depending on where we dropped anchor, we always stretched, meditated, worked out, and explored on foot.

By the end of the trip, my boat mates were *asking* for exercise.

Many of my clients have told me similar stories of their transformed vacations. Danny Meyer, owner of four restaurants including the prestigious Union Square Café, spent most of his vacation time lounging on the beach while basking in the sun as he watched the porpoises in the water.

Then he tried something different. He played tennis for hours every day. He didn't even think about sitting on the beach until the last day. And even then, he vegged for only an hour.

I'm not saying that you shouldn't rest on your vacation. To nurture a Sound mind, I strongly encourage rest and meditation. But I also suggest fitness and healthy eating.

It's my firm belief that most people gain weight on vacation because they are bored. They eat junk because they have nothing better to do. I'm going to help you design each day so that you are never bored. Here's a sample schedule.

Sunrise. Although it is not mandatory, I like to start and end my day with the sun. There's just something spiritual about it. And there's also something nice about not paying too much attention to my watch.

Stretch and sit quietly for morning meditation. The art of breathing is one that is lost on most of us during our fast-paced days. After your meditation, do some form of exercise—a power walk, a swim, a run, or a series of calisthenics. After your exercise session, stretch and finish with some abdominal work.

Early morning. Fix a nutritious breakfast and rest while you digest. Read that book you've never gotten around to. Watch the waves. Listen to the birds.

Midmorning. Depending on where you are, spend the next few hours sightseeing either on foot or by pedal. If you're at Disney World, walk through Epcot Center. If you're at Club Med, go for a long walk on the beach. If you're in Paris, cycle along the Seine. If you're in Athens, walk through La Placa. Wherever you are, make your way around without using a motorized vehicle.

Noon. Eat your largest meal of the day.

Early afternoon. Rest.

Midafternoon. Do something fun and active, such as playing touch foot-

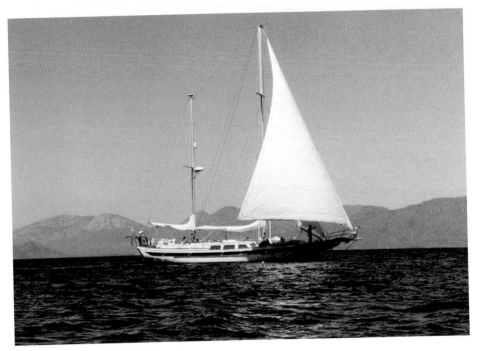

Sailing in the Greek Isles

ball or paddleball on the beach, perfecting handstands in the pool, surfing the waves, inline skating in a park, or combing the beach for shells. (Shell searching is one of my favorite activities.)

Early evening. Eat a small meal.

That schedule will give you 6 to 8 hours of physical activity. Yet only the aerobic and strength-training exercise in the morning will feel like exercise. The rest will just seem like part of the day. And best of all, you'll return fitter, more toned, and probably slimmer than when you left. I know many of my clients did. "My husband and I both lost weight. We both felt good, and yet we also had a holiday," said one of my clients, who in the past had used her vacations as an excuse to toss aside her Sound eating and exercise habits.

And you don't have to feel deprived. You can celebrate and you can indulge. Just keep your indulgences Sound. For example, when one of my clients went to Club Med, she knew the Club served delicious bread. On the last day of her trip, she allowed herself to have a piece of bread. And she felt good about herself.

Sundown to sunrise. Rest, meditate, and sleep. As much as we try, most of us don't get enough sleep day in and day out, so this is your first priority for vacation.

Here are some tips for planning a Sound vacation.

Pick your vacation mates carefully. Don't automatically think your family and good friends are the best companions for your fitness vacation. If they don't already exercise and eat Soundly, they'll complain the whole time, throwing you off track. You want to vacation with people of similar fitness abilities and backgrounds. For example, couples usually do better with couples, and singles with singles.

Do some homework. After reading the Sound Eating chapter, you should already be armed with the knowledge to eat Soundly at any restaurant during your vacation. You could literally eat at a burger-chain restaurant every day and still stay healthy. But do you really want to eat that, or would you rather try out the local ethnic fare? I know I would rather have the latter. Do some homework on the Internet and with your travel agent beforehand so you're already familiar with the restaurants, menus, and delicacies in your vacation spot.

For example, by planning ahead, you'll learn that you can survive your trip to Italy without turning into a "carb face." All of the Mediterranean countries, from Italy to Greece, serve great fish dishes. Order them.

What if you don't have time to do your homework? Then do some active homework on the first day of your vacation by walking around town and looking at the menus of the various eateries. Befriending the concierge at the hotel might not be a bad idea either. Just be forewarned that they don't always have the best health sensibilities.

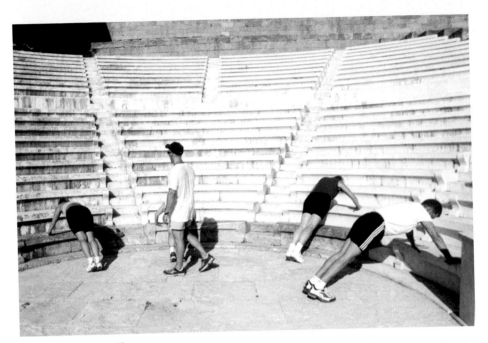

A fitness vacation in Europe

Search out scenery. You don't have to go all the way to the Greek Islands to spend a wonderfully beautiful vacation. You can probably find some scenic spots within hours of your house. But do make scenery a top priority. There's nothing like the sun sparkling off water or the mountaintops to inspire quiet meditation.

SURVIVING A CHANGE IN HEALTH

It's no surprise that health problems rank within the top 10 reasons people fall off their fitness wagons. Whether you have back pain or have been diag-nosed with a chronic disease, you'll need to plan carefully to ensure a Sound future.

Sound Eating, Training, Thinking, and Living habits are even more important if you have a chronic disease such as diabetes, cancer, heart disease, or AIDS. Your mind is incredibly powerful and can see you through the gravest of situations. Physical exercise and proper nutrition have been shown to increase one's physical and mental awareness, improve overall health, lower blood cholesterol, lower blood pressure, strengthen weak and deteriorating hearts, and reverse the effects of wasting in both cancer and AIDS patients.

Sound Eating, Training, Thinking, and Living make up the greatest holistic line of defense your body has. You must work hand-in-hand with your physician during this process. Tell your doctor about the supplements you are taking and the exercises you're performing. Allow your doctor to suggest modifications. Explore alternative medicine, but don't ignore conventional medicine.

Always listen to your body. Pain has no place in an exercise routine. If you feel discomfort, you are either doing an exercise incorrectly or you need to modify the exercise for your specific body type and size. Throughout my Sound Training chapter, I offer numerous tips on how to do this. But the best way to learn how to push yourself to the limit—and no further—is by honing your mind-body connection.

Anything from medication side effects and the disease itself to depression about the disease can lower your energy levels. Your strength will change from day to day. Don't berate yourself because you could do 20 pushups on Monday but only 5 on Wednesday.

Embrace spirituality. I won't tell you that chronic disease strikes for a reason. But once it does strike, you can deal with it in one of two ways. You can sulk and feel like a victim, or you can search for a hidden meaning and learn what you can from the disease. Spend some time alone and contemplate how the disease can teach you something new about life. No matter what happens, never stop fighting. Do everything you can do to beat your disease. That means exercising, sleeping, lowering stress, eating better, and taking vitamins.

A SOUND PREGNANCY

There's nothing like change to throw off a fitness program, and one of the biggest life changes is pregnancy. But just because a baby is on the way doesn't mean you need to spend the rest of your life losing your baby weight.

You can start by not gaining it. Of course, you do want to gain the amount of weight prescribed by your doctor. Don't starve yourself, and once you get the go-ahead from your doctor, continue your Sound Mind, Sound Body program.

Gone are the days when doctors told women to stop exercising once they became pregnant. Now doctors say that women—assuming it's an uneventful pregnancy—can continue doing whatever form of exercise they were doing before pregnancy. In fact, staying fit throughout your pregnancy increases the chances of having a sound delivery and recovery.

◆ Only do exercises that you were doing before you were pregnant. If you're pregnant and thinking about starting a new fitness program, consult with your obstetrician/gynecologist first.

◆ After your first trimester, don't do anything in a prone position, such as Crunches. This can put pressure on one of the main blood vessels leading to your uterus, cutting off your baby's oxygen supply.

◆ Exercise at what feels like a moderate level. Pay attention to your maximum perceived rate of exertion (MPRE).

After you've had the baby, you can start resuming your fitness routine in about 6 weeks, depending on your delivery. Talk to your doctor about your plans. Start with cardiovascular exercise. When that feels good, return to your weight-lifting routine, paying particular attention to Reverse Crunches to pull your abdominal area back in.

The 10-Step Pregnancy Shape-Up

Women fear losing their abs, hips, butt, and triceps during pregnancy. The pregnancy program I recommend focuses on these areas and produces fantastic results. The exercises remain the same throughout the pregnancy, except for eliminating prone exercises (including Crunches) after the first trimester. Before trying this program, get medical clearance from your doctor.

1. Good Mornings (p. 81)
2. Basic Crunches (p. 101)*, Bicycles (p. 110), and Reverse Crunches (p. 103)
3. David's Isometric Abs (p. 108), done while seated and while standing by contracting the abdominal muscles
4. Plié Squats and Plié Squats with Calf Raises (p. 55)
5. Stiff-Leg Dead Lifts (p. 57) and Partial Dead Lifts (p. 58)
6. Reverse Lunges with Crossover Lunges (p. 66)
7. Deluxe Pushup Routine (p. 46)
8. Dips on a Bench (p. 97) with Reverse-Grip Pushups (p. 99)
9. One-Arm Dumbbell Rows (p. 76) with Pullovers (p. 79)*
10. Walking Alexandra Lunges (p. 66)

*After the first trimester, do not do Crunches or Pullovers. Instead, you can work your abs by sitting on the edge of a bench, raising your feet from the floor, and performing slow leg rotations.

YOUR BACKYARD
BOOT CAMP

One of the best ways to bring your friends into your new wellness fold is to hold your own backyard boot camp. When they hear these two words, many people think of the army, with a drill sergeant and maybe an oppressive atmosphere. That's not what I'm suggesting.

I'm talking about a wellness party, where you push yourself and your friends slightly past your limits. More often than not, we are too easy on ourselves when we exercise alone. But boot camp provides the motivation to push to that next level. Boot camp is about discovering your physical, psychological, and emotional limitations and moving beyond them.

Yet this isn't about pain or oppression or bossing your friends around. (Or at least it doesn't have to be.) Consider holding a tranquillity boot camp. The idea of a serene boot camp might seem like an oxymoron, but it's one of the best ways to mesh your Sound Thinking with your Sound Training and Sound Eating. And it's exactly what will draw your friends into your new Sound lifestyle.

I've organized and acted as drill sergeant at a number of boot camps in the Hamptons, on lavish estate grounds, and even in Central Park. For a true tranquillity boot camp, I like to organize the day around the sun. I start at sunrise with some stretching and meditation, and then move into some cardiovascular exercise, whether it's a cardio sculpting routine or a power walk.

After some cardio, we cool down and stretch. Then I serve a healthy breakfast such as protein shakes or an egg frittata. After breakfast, I usually allow the boot campers to spend quality time together talking and laughing as they digest. Then I move into more hard-core strength moves such as pushups, squat thrusts, and, depending on the location, mountain climbing, swimming, and so on. After that, we spend some quiet time in meditation.

You don't need to hold your boot camp in a posh location for it to be a success. You can do it in your own backyard or a nearby park. Here are some Sound boot camp tips.

Pick a theme. An upcoming event in your life may dictate the theme. For example, if you or a friend is getting married, then you can hold a bridal boot camp. If summer is approaching, you might hold a bikini boot camp. (See "Heidi Klum's Bikini Boot Camp" on page 228.) If you and your friends play the same sport, you might hold a season fitness blastoff camp. Whatever theme you pick, make the most of it. For a bikini boot camp, have everyone show up in their bikinis. There's nothing like reality staring you in the face to encourage you to get in a good workout.

Your theme will partially direct your weight-lifting moves. If you're toning your back for a low-cut wedding dress, you'll definitely want to work in some dumbbell rows. If you're getting ready for bikini belly weather, then crunches are a must. Jumping jacks, pushups, squats, lunges, running in place, and squat thrusts are also nice to throw in as well as any of my signature moves.

Choose your friends carefully. Yes, you do want your Sound teachings to rub off on your friends, but you also want your camp to run without a hitch. Invite guests with like interests and similar fitness abilities. Keep your invitation list to no more than six people. I've found that any more than that tends to produce whining. Smaller groups are also much more conducive to balancing physical energy with spirituality. Remember: You don't want to turn your boot camp into an '80s-era aerobics class.

Cater to your friends' interests. When designing the camp, think about what you and your friends enjoy doing together. If you often dance at nightclubs, consider making dancing part of your day. If you all love Latin music, play it. And if you're all sun goddesses, work in some time to worship the sun. (Just make sure to wear sunscreen!) If you're spa girls, hire a massage therapist, pedicurist, or facial expert for a portion of the day.

Know their fitness levels. You don't want to make your boot camp so hard that your friends quit halfway through the day. Yet you don't want to make it so easy that you don't challenge them. Push their comfort levels, but don't leave anyone behind.

Make it BYODB. That is, bring your own dumbbells. When you send out the invitations, make sure to let them know what to bring: cross-training shoes, dumbbells, a change of clothes, and a towel.

Provide sustenance. Offer plenty of water and some food between exercise sessions. Serve pears, apples, and berries. Offer protein shakes (see page 193), frittatas (see page 167), and low-carbohydrate energy bars.

Use your natural surroundings. The makeup of your backyard will influence your choice of activities. If you have a pool, use it to swim laps, tread water, or play water polo. If you have hills, do a series of hill repeats with running or power hiking. Make sure to clean up your yard ahead of time. You don't want anyone tripping over a sprinkler or stepping in dog doo.

Take a field trip. For your meditation, go somewhere scenic or fun. I believe that each person can find inner peace without coaching. So don't feel the need to coach your friends through a meditation. Just take them to a playground, a lake, or even a carousel to watch the goings-on and let them get deep inside their own heads. Then power walk home.

Have some fun. My most successful boot camps include a good amount of exercise, some healthy eating, and a dose of partying. Life isn't black and white, and neither is your boot camp. At the very worst, partying will give you a reason to exercise. Feel empowered, not guilty.

Heidi Klum's Bikini Boot Camp

START YOUR WORKOUT with some light stretches, including Good Mornings and Good Mornings with Knee Bends.

Death, taxes, and Heidi Klum's incredible physical and spiritual beauty are three givens in the world today. But as hard as it may be to believe, even Heidi came to me with a pet peeve. She thought her butt and thighs needed a lift. Clearly, God blessed her with an amazing face and torso, but her concern was with defying gravity down below.

That's why I designed the following boot camp blast for her. It helped her create an amazing body for her *Sports Illustrated* swimsuit issue photo shoot. Now I'm not saying that this workout will make you look like Heidi. (And as you remember from chapter 2, you don't want to look like her anyway.) But it *will* help you look like an improved you.

Because of her nonstop schedule, Heidi's time with me was sporadic and limited. When on the road, she didn't always have access to a gym or weights. But the following workout kept her fit wherever she was. Use it for your backyard boot camp, or use it to keep fit in your office or while on vacation.

Run through the routine on page 230 once with very light weight or no weight at all.

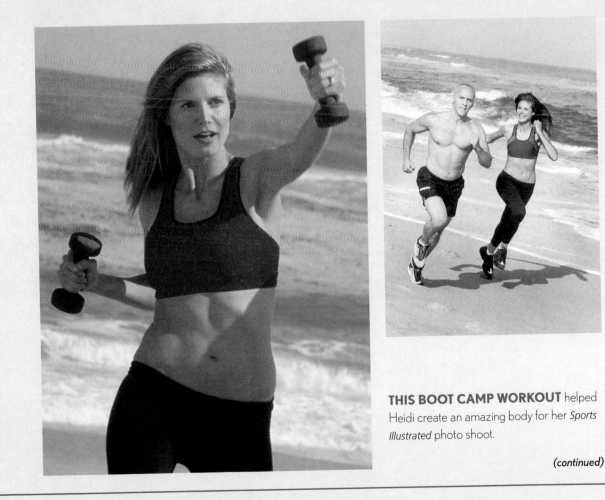

THIS BOOT CAMP WORKOUT helped Heidi create an amazing body for her *Sports Illustrated* photo shoot.

(continued)

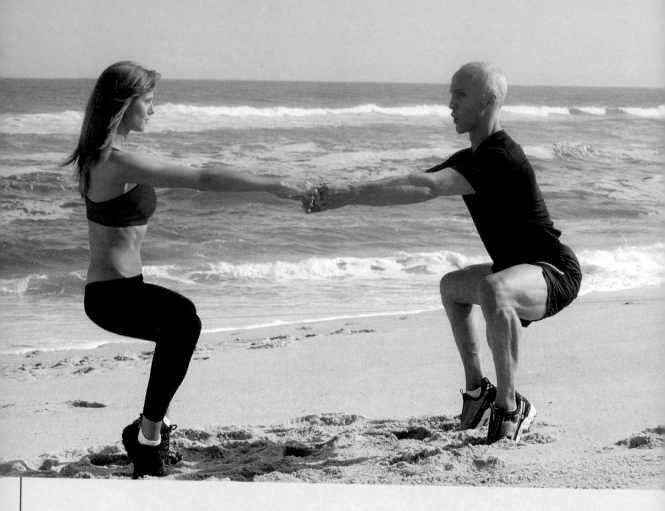

Heidi Klum's Bikini Boot Camp (cont.)

◆ 2 minutes: Light stretching, including Good Mornings and Good Mornings with Knee Bends

◆ 1 minute: Jumping Jacks

◆ 30 seconds: David's Platypus Walks

◆ 1 minute: Shadowboxing with Crossovers, Uppercuts, and Knee Bends

◆ 1 minute: Plié Squats with Calf Raises

◆ 2 minutes: Reverse Lunges with Side Kicks

◆ 1 minute: Squat Thrusts

◆ 1 minute: Scissors Reverse Crunches

◆ 2 minutes: David's Donkey Deluxe

◆ 1 minute: Bench Stepups (if possible) with Triceps Kickbacks

◆ 1 minute: Pushups

Take a 2- to 3-minute rest and hydration break and run through the routine again. Then repeat the whole sequence two to four more times with ankle weights and dumbbells if you have them with you. The entire program should last 45 minutes to an hour and a half.

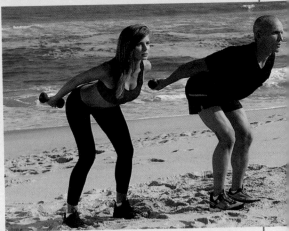

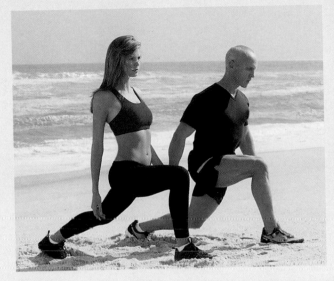

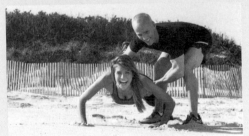

THESE EXERCISES target all of Heidi's major muscles, including her chest, back, arms, abs, glutes, and legs.

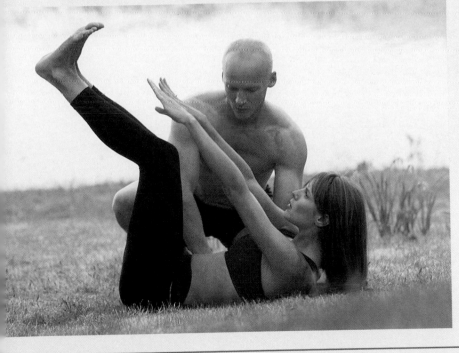

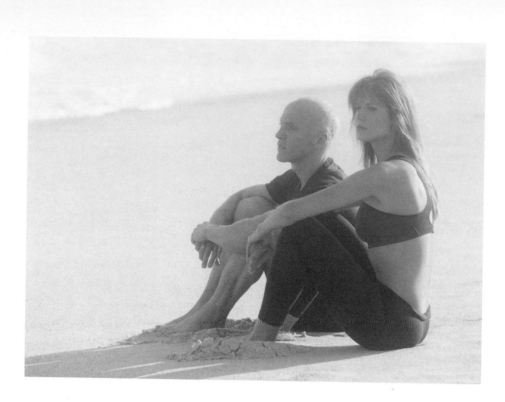

RECONNECTING
WITH YOUR INNER SPIRIT

I'm sure that you are pleased with the new answers to your self-test. I would like to share with you a very personal moment. As I discussed earlier in the book, wellness is a total-body concept—mental, physical, psychological, and spiritual. The search for the proper balance is encountered on the "road," and upon successful completion of your journey, the proper balance is established. For me, finding balance meant finding time to give back to the community. My grandmother taught me that God gave us two hands—one to receive, but the other, more important, to give. I took that lesson to heart, and when I was asked to participate in a 575-mile, 7-day bicycle marathon through the mountains of Montana to raise money for research for an AIDS vaccine, I jumped at the opportunity.

I faced many challenges—both psychological and physical—over the course of those 7 days. But with the help of a group of guys that I cycled with—we called ourselves Team Alliance—we met, faced, and conquered our fears and challenges Soundly.

Your Wellness Quotient Retest

Remember the self-test you took in chapter 2? Are you ready to see how much progress you've made during the past 6 weeks? Let's do it. Compare your answers here to the answers your wrote down 6 weeks ago.

1. How do you see yourself now? How do you believe other people perceive you physically? Hopefully, your self-confidence grew during the past 6 weeks as people complimented you on your appearance and vitality.

2. What were your goals for this program? What are they now? At some point during the past 6 weeks, you probably experienced the realization that your true goals had more to do with pushing yourself to your fullest potential and less to do with looking like a model or actress.

3. How has your attitude toward food changed? You probably look at doughnuts and other foods in a completely different way than you did before week 1. You now have better reasons to forgo the doughnut than mere calories. Good health, better energy, and feeling and looking better all contribute to your willpower and motivation.

4. What is your attitude toward exercise now? Exercise probably isn't something you have to force yourself to do—it's a challenge that you tackle with your mind and your body.

5. How has your attitude toward life changed? Your world is hopefully much brighter and filled with more possibilities than it was 6 weeks ago.

Throughout my training, I have had to reconnect to my core—my inner spirit, if you will. In the end, that is what we ultimately rely upon when the going gets tough. On July 15, 2001, I took on my biggest physical challenge to date—my first century ride. (For those of you who think I'm referring to the 21st century, it is actually the lingo for a 100-mile bicycle ride.) Following a beach boot camp, I met up with my friend, Will, and at 8:30 A.M., we were off, armed with plenty of water, Clif bars, and Gu. Miles 1 through 60 were a bit of a blur and went rather quickly—we were making a quick pit stop in 2 hours and 53 minutes. I thought it was going to be a breeze! Boy, was I wrong! Miles 60 through 80 were the longest miles I had ever experienced on my bicycle. I didn't think I was going to make it. I was angry, sore, and disillusioned (sound familiar?). Even fitness gurus have their moments, and I was definitely having mine.

I finally started talking to myself at

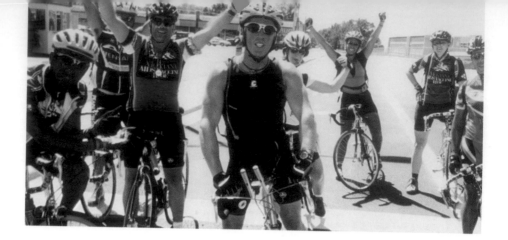

around mile 75, convincing myself that it was all going to be good. I can remember saying out loud, "Look, you're going to do this thing anyway, so which will it be—easy or hard?" At that instant, I felt my body and muscles relaxing. I regained control of my breathing. All of the negative energy that had been building up inside my body and mixing with the lactic acid was coming to the surface. I knew that if I stuck out the next few miles, I would complete what I had set out to do.

My riding partner had to quit at mile 80 because he was late for work. He asked if I was going to continue, to which I incredulously answered, "Of course!"

By mile 92, I was singing again—I felt that I was becoming one with my body. I had almost lost control 30 miles back, but was able to quickly regain my composure. Then, at mile 98.9, the inexplicable happened. Something caused me to look heavenward, and I burst into uncontrollable

tears. Elation? Exhaustion? Temporary mental breakdown? Only passing the bar exam had ever made me feel that way. I was so proud of myself. I had taken on a seemingly insurmountable challenge, allowed it to almost get the better of me, and ultimately defeated my demons and prevailed. In that instant, I hit the mark and emerged virtuous and victorious.

You don't necessarily need to complete a 100-mile bicycle ride to mark your successful journey to wellness. Your demons may be otherwise masked. But please take the lessons gleaned from my experiences to heart. To succeed after 6 weeks, you might begin to see life the way the ancient Greeks viewed the world: Virtue is hitting the mark; sin is missing the mark. Pushing yourself to your fullest potential is your greatest reward in this lifelong journey to wellness. Eating better, living longer, and taking care of yourself have now become your ultimate prizes.

ACKNOWLEDGMENTS

Dad—Your strength, integrity, and devotion to wellness have always been a major inspiration to me. It all began in the basement with a pair of old dumbbells. Who could have imagined it would lead to this? With deepest love, pride, and respect.

Mom—From the beginning, our hearts and souls have always been connected. With your love and support, anything is possible. "Am I a gentleman yet?"

Bonnie—Without you, none of this would be possible. You free my heart and soul to feel, create, and be. I love you so much.

Stacie—Thank you for your love and support. With your genius, we've created the MS2 Spa Collection, and I'm very proud and appreciative of all of your efforts.

Elise—For always keeping me informed of my 4-star days. Your love helped get me through some dark days.

Elie—For your endless devotion and tireless work, I am eternally grateful.

Marcy—You enhance my life—my love, appreciation, friendship, and devotion to you always.

Desiree—For always speaking your heart's truth and for being the most levelheaded Cancer I know—thank you for your love and support. It is returned in kind.

Heidi—A thousand kisses for your friendship, love, and generosity of spirit. Your participation in this book enriched it immeasurably. I am eternally grateful.

Chava, Sidney, Samantha, and Cara—With you, there is promise and hope for a better tomorrow. I love you all and am so very proud of you.

Poppa, Grandma, Aunt Shelley, and Uncle Sidney—I love and miss you all. I feel blessed having so many angels taking care of me.

Marc—You taught me the importance of making the most of life.

Jamie—My friend—thanks for listening when I needed an ear. Through your strength and courage, I have learned so much. You are truly an inspiration and I love you.

Shonna—For being able to look into my eyes and capture my soul. I am so proud of your work. With love.

Stephanie, Rich, Chris, Jim, Kelly, Donna, and the team at Rodale—Thank you for making my first book experience so fulfilling. I really appreciate the time, patience, and attention you all took to be true to the integrity of my voice. I am very proud of our collaborative effort.

Alisa—For helping me articulate my vision, passion, and journey. I look forward to working with you again and again and again.

Ed, Laura, Teril, Kendra, Danielle, Jim, and the sales team at Henri Bendel—Thank you for including me in your family.

Team Alliance—For helping to teach me the importance of the team over self—"We own Montana!"

Rich and the team at Gym Source—To the best exercise equipment center in the world, thanks for everything. You help make the Madison Square Club the state-of-the-art facility it is today.

Chris—To my unofficial editor—your voice and sound reason resonates throughout—I feel privileged to count you among my friends (and advisers).

Catherine—You were the first to see the possibility of it all. Thank you for believing in me. I love you.

To my trainers and staff at the Madison Square Club—You're the best, simply the best.

To all my friends whom I have failed to list (and you know who you are)—I thank you for your support and love not only throughout the process of writing this book but also in all of my endeavors. I am able to give love because I am surrounded by so much love.

To all of my clients—I thank you for enriching my life. This book is a reflection and collection of my life's experiences, which you have all played a major part in developing. I hope you are as proud of my accomplishment as I am of all of yours.

Chris and Ardelia—Thank you for transforming my recipes into delicious and nutritious delights. You have helped make the One of a Kind Food program the success it is and something we are all very proud of.

Linda W.—When I needed advice and counsel, you were there to make sense of it all. I am proud to have you as one of my clients and privileged to consider you one of my friends.

Jennifer and Alan—Lots of love and gratitude for all your help. I couldn't have done it without you. From recipe testing to one-finger typing, nobody does it better!

Donald—Many thanks for providing me with the space to create and expand the Madison Square Club.